Preparation for Pregnancy is the passport to positive health for the new millennium. The FORESIGHT strategy pulls together a wealth of international research and moulds it into a practical programme for health enhancement prior to conception.

By optimising the health of the sperm, ova and uterus, it is ensured that new life springs from a basis of strength and vitality. A bibliography of 555 scientific references gives validation.

Nutrition in the broadest sense; the avoidance of smoking, alcohol and drugs; non-invasive contraception; genito-urinary and other infections; allergy, malabsorption and infestation; essential trace elements; heavy metals and other environmental toxins are fully covered. A protocol is outlined for the setting up of a Preconception Clinic.

Recent FORESIGHT research has shown 327 consecutive pregnancies without a miscarriage, stillbirth or malformation. No baby was born underweight. None were admitted to a Special Care Baby Unit. 86% of those parents with infertility problems had given birth by the end of the study.

The modern practitioner who wishes to spare his/her patients the agony of childlessness or a sad outcome to a pregnancy and to bring instead the joy and fulfilment of a healthy baby should read this book.

Suzanne Gail Bradley is a social worker and teacher with a special interest in health matters. She is the author of numerous articles and papers on the importance of diet.

PREPARATION

for

PREGNANCY

AN ESSENTIAL GUIDE

*International research
into preconceptual health and pregnancy outcome including
the* FORESIGHT *experience*

Suzanne Gail Bradley
&
Nicholas Bennett
with contributions from
Dr Damien Downing, Dr Belinda Dawes and Mrs Belinda Barnes

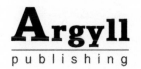

Argyll
publishing

First Published 1995
Paperback edition 1997
Argyll Publishing
Glendaruel
Argyll PA22 3AE
Scotland

British Library Cataloguing-in-Publication Data.
A catalogue record for this book is available from the British Library.

ISBN 1 874640 73 4

Origination
Cordfall Ltd, Glasgow

Printing
ColourBooks Ltd, Dublin

Contents

Preface

A fact well-known among those who breed racehorses, champion dogs, cattle and other animals is that the best outcome is achievable when the health and vigour of both prospective parents are optimal at the time of conception. Yet with breeding human beings, who with typical hubris we seem to regard as above mere animals, the whole thing is left to chance.

Why is this? Cynics might suggest that racehorses etc can have a high cash value whereas human babies have less quantifiable value.

Whatever the reason – and sheer ignorance must play a part – it is a serious reflection on health professionals that an initiative to remedy this state of affairs had to come initially from the essentially lay charity FORESIGHT and its farsighted founder, Belinda Barnes.

FORESIGHT has wisely emphasised the importance of care prior to conception and the role of genotoxins, although defective nutrition and/or exposure to fetotoxins in utero are increasingly being recognised as additional risk factors. For example, the fetal alcohol syndrome (FAS) caused by the mother drinking alcohol during pregnancy was only officially recognised by the mainstream medical profession some twenty years ago, although a reference can be found to it in the Bible. (Judges 13, v14)

This is not exactly a triumph of medical diagnosis. Warnings of the dangers to the unborn child from mothers' smoking are now common on the walls of doctors' surgeries and antenatal clinics, but there is still no law and only mild social disapproval, to forbid this particular form of 'baby bashing'.

Of nutritional disorders, the role of folate deficiency in spina bifida has at last been officially recognised. So pregnant mothers should be advised to 'eat up their greens' and maybe also the folate supplement. But, dear reader, do not rejoice prematurely, for a 1991 'expert' report from the Department of Health indicated that there is no need for any mineral nutritional supplements during pregnancy, even iron!

It has recently come to light that a low birth weight is itself one of the risk factors for the development of some major disorders in later life, including hypertension, heart disease and diabetes. Since nutritional and toxic factors predispose towards a low birth weight, they acquire special importance.

The information in this book is relevant to two more general matters. Firstly, the earliest developmental stages at which an organism is damaged tend to be those most highly geared to adverse longer term consequences. Secondly, any species that tends to neglect the welfare of its descendants tends also to damage its own evolutionary survival prospects. We have heard and maybe laughed at the cynical jest, "Why should I worry about posterity: what has posterity ever done for me?"

What can we do in the face of such cynicism, indifference and what appears to be woeful ignorance in some quarters? Perhaps the health authorities should provide schools with posters and leaflets setting out the FORESIGHT principles. More preconception clinics need to be set up, preferably with help from the Department of Health, so that more babies born in future will have a better chance to achieve their true genetic potential. But the most important need is for more education on preconception and prenatal care. I therefore recommend that all concerned should read, mark, learn and inwardly digest the practical information and advice in this important book.

Professor D Bryce-Smith
University of Reading

Introduction

A primary desire of mankind is to have children. In fact our future human existence is directly related to the health and well-being of our offspring. For many couples pregnancy and the birth of a healthy child is a time of great fulfilment and happiness. However, in our modern society there is an ever increasing number of couples who are confronted with unexplained infertility problems, or the experience of a previous pregnancy which resulted in miscarriage, stillbirth, malformation, or impaired foetal development. Medical and scientific research is constantly evaluating the factors that can contribute to these problems. In many cases the use of specialised tests in the preconceptual period or during pregnancy have improved fertility status, the rate of conception, and the diagnosis of foetal abnormalities. Amniocentesis, ultrasound scanning, and hormonal tests of the woman's blood or urine are regularly used to confirm both normal placental function and foetal development.

In recent years scientific evidence has also indicated that genetic, microbiological, biochemical, dietary, and environmental factors play a major role in affecting fertility and foetal outcome. FORESIGHT research in my laboratory has shown that foetal development can be strongly dependent on the status of the pregnant mother with respect to various essential and toxic trace elements. Examples of the most important essential trace elements are calcium, magnesium, iron, selenium, copper, and zinc; and toxic trace elements are lead, cadmium, and mercury. In general before and throughout pregnancy there is an important balance between having optimum levels of essential trace elements relative to very low levels of toxic trace elements. Major factors which influence this balance are smoking activity (active and passive), alcohol consumption, use of the contraceptive pill, exposure to some pesticides and nitrates, food additives, inadequate dietary status, and poor food quality consumption. Moreover, analysis of maternal and neonatal tissues and fluids, especially placental material has shown that abnormally high lead and/or cadmium levels in conjunction with low zinc can contribute to human stillbirths and foetal malformations.

Research combined with experience acquired by the ever increasing number of successful FORESIGHT pregnancies for couples with previous infertility or pregnancy problems has shown that the future health status of a child starts at the preconceptual period. As a farmer's son my father always made it clear to me that it is vital to prepare and nourish the soil carefully before planting any seeds. In fact a good crop is the combination of many factors. The same is true of pregnancy. This is what makes the FORESIGHT approach in planning for a healthy baby such an important guide. It addresses a basic plan for both partners, recognising that natural family planning, combined with a strong awareness of dietary, environmental, and social factors is vital before conception. For those cases where clinical and medical testing shows an imbalance in nutritional status, excessive smoking and/or alcohol consumption, genito-urinary infections, allergies, candida or other intestinal infestation problems, the FORESIGHT programme aims to correct or eliminate these factors.

A recently published report on pregnancy outcomes achieved by 367 couples who had been enrolled on a FORESIGHT preconception programme during 1990–92 showed that 89% of the women (327) had become pregnant and 327 healthy children had been born. These impressive statistics relate to a majority of cases where there had been a previous history of reproductive problems, infertility, or multi-miscarriages, stillbirths, low birthweights, or malformations. It is hoped that this book will provide factual information for the interested professional on the FORESIGHT approach and result in many more healthy children.

Dr Neil I Ward BSc, MSc(Hons), PhD

Ward, NI, Watson, R, Bryce-Smith, D (1987) Placental element levels in relation to fetal development for obstetrically 'normal' births: A study of 37 elements, evidence for effects of cadmium, lead, and zinc on fetal growth, and for smoking as a source of cadmium. Int J Biosocial Research 9(1), 63-81

Ward, NI, Durrant, S, Sankey, RJ, Bound, JP, Bryce-Smith, D (1990) Elemental factors in human fetal development. J Nutritional Medicine, 1, 19-26

Ward, NI. , Bryce-Smith, D (1993). Lead, cadmium, and zinc levels in relation to fetal development and abnormalities (stillbirths, spina bifida, and hydrocephalus). Heavy Metals in the Environment, Vol 2, Allan, RJ, Nriagu, JO (eds.), CEP Consultants Ltd, Edinburgh, 280-284

Ward, NI (1995) Preconceptional care and pregnancy outcome. J Nutritional and Environmental Medicine, 5, 205-208

Preconceptual Care
and Pregnancy Outcome

Letter to the Editors of the
Journal of Nutritional & Environmental Medicine (1995)

Sirs: We would like to report the pregnancy outcomes achieved by 367 couples, average ages 34 (22–45) for females and 36 (25–59) for males, who had been enrolled on a FORESIGHT[1] preconception programme during 1990–92. FORESIGHT clinicians completed investigations of both partners which included questionnaires, analysis of essential nutrient status in blood, hair and/or sweat, and semen analysis. Common, but often symptomless, genito-urinary infections were sought by testing endocervical swabs, urine and post-prostatic massage secretions while blood was tested for chlamydial antibodies to diagnose active pelvic inflammatory disease.[2, 3]

Data evaluation showed that 90% of males and 60% of females regularly drank alcohol while 45% of the men but 57% of the women smoked.

Among the 367 couples, 217 (59%) had a previous history of reproductive problems; 136 (37%) had suffered from infertility (for <1 to >10years) and 139 (38%) had histories of from one to five previous miscarriages; 11 (3%) had given birth to a stillborn child, 40 were small-for-dates and 15 were of low birthweight (<2500g); 7 were malformed and 3 infants died of sudden infant death syndrome. A total of 86 females reported more than one of these problems. Of the male partners, 154 (42%) had a semen analysis because of infertility and most had a reduction in sperm quality. Commonest complaints among prospective parents were fatigue, headaches/migraines, cold feet, back pain, abdominal bloating and constipation.

Written and telephone follow-ups carried out in 1993 revealed that 327 (89%) of the women had become pregnant and 327 children had been born since enrolment. There were no multiple pregnancies. In remarkable contrast to the couples' previous experience, all their babies (137 males and 190 females) were born healthy and were well developed at birth which occurred from 36 to 41 weeks (mean 38.5 weeks). Average birthweight was 3265g (2368–4145). None were malformed and none were transferred to special care baby units. Among 204 couples with infertility problems, 175 (86%) had achieved healthy pregnancies.

Neil Ward PhD
Director of Research
Dept of Chemistry
University of Surrey

With acknowledgement to the following doctors who participated in the study.
Dr Marilyn Glenville BEd MA PhD Dip EHP NLP;
Dr Ellen Grant MB ChB DObst RCOG;
Dr Jonathan Hardy MA BM MF HOM;
Dr Tom Hayes MA MB BC HIR DR COG MRC GP;
Dr Patrick Kingsley MB BS MRCS LRCP DObst RCOG;
Dr J Meldrum MB ChB DCH DA BObst RCOG MRCGP HTD;
Dr Jenny Nevison MB BS;
Dr M Nightingale MB BS MRCGP FFDRCS MRCS LRCP;
Dr Patricia Sankey MB ChB MRCGD DObst RCOG;
Dr C Scott-Moncrieff MB ChB MFH OM;
Dr Pamela Tatham MB BS (London);
Dr K Thorley MA MB BChir MRC GP DRCOG.

1 Barnes B, Grant E, Mumby K et al, Nutrition and preconception care. Lancet 1985; i: 1297
2 Barnes B, Bradley SG, Planning for a Healthy Baby. London: Edbury Press 1990
3 Grant ECG, Sexual Chemistry. London: Cedar, Reed Books 1994

SECTION ONE

1 THE NECESSITY FOR PREGNANCY PREPARATION

2 SETTING UP A CLINIC

3 PRECONCEPTION MEDICAL CHECKS
– THE FORESIGHT WAY

SECTION ONE

1 The Necessity for Pregnancy Preparation

"I know of nothing so potent in maintaining good health in laboratory animals as perfectly constituted food; I know of nothing so potent in producing ill-health as improperly constituted food. This, too, is the experience of stockbreeders. Is man an exception to the rule so universally applicable to the higher animals?"

(McCarrison 1984)

The FORESIGHT approach advocated in this book is based on the same principles adopted by farmers, race-horse breeders and zoos, all of whom supply their breeding animals with individual, precise nutritional requirements to ensure optimum health. It also draws on the multitude of research on other factors which adversely affect health, including pollutants and infections.

Preconception care is not a new concept. Not only can advice be found in the Bible (Judges), it abounds in the many traditions passed down through generations, and is sometimes relegated to the status of "old wives' tales". The Masai tribe had specific times for marriage to ensure that the bride had had a few months on a highly nutritious diet. Sometimes the preparation was extended to the father-to-be as well. (Price 1945) Work on animals has confirmed the wisdom of these practices and it is well known in zoos that if animals are to breed successfully they need the right nutrition, as part of a programme aiming for optimum health. (Hoffer 1983)

Do doctors need to be concerned about pregnancy preparation? Perhaps that question is answered by a doctor, Hamish Sutherland of the Department of Obstetrics and Gynaecology, University of Aberdeen in a letter to the Lancet in 1982:

> Too many women make their first antenatal visit with the pregnancy already compromised or at risk from smoking, inappropriate nutrition, ingestion of a variety of pharmaceutical preparations (including oral contraceptive steroids), genito-urinary infection, anaemia, and poor dental hygiene. All too frequently cervical cytology and rubella immunity status are unknown.
>
> *(Sutherland 1982)*

In addition to the dangers to the fetus and child that he mentions one can add others, including increasing air and water pollution, increasing radiation from both non-ionising and ionising sources, greater use of chemicals in the workplace and home, all of which result in adverse pregnancy outcomes that are avoidable, given the knowledge that is available to those who seek it.

There is, unfortunately, too much evidence to show that pregnancy preparation is not treated seriously by everyone. There will, of course, always be unplanned pregnancies and problem pregnancies, but the research shows that many could be avoided. (Adams 1993) Where pregnancy is a planned event with good preparation the incidence of problem pregnancies is reduced to a much lower figure. (Ward 1993) Social and economic situations are certainly factors. In Britain, data shows that the lower the social class, the lower the income and the further north, the greater is the risk of poor health generally, including fetal and child health. (Black 1982) Deprivation has been linked with low birth weight and children's heights. (Reading 1993)

Assessing the total incidence of problem pregnancies is almost impossible. Research has shown that prenatal damage may not be revealed for many years. (Holiverda-Kuipers 1987) Dutch research has shown that if a woman is deprived of food around the time of conception, while she may give birth to a child of normal birth weight, that child's own baby is at high risk of being a low birth weight child. (Lumley 1992) Even those outcomes which are known are not always recorded. No-one knows the incidence of epilepsy, dyslexia or behavioural problems.The incidence of miscarriage will never be certain, though the statistics would suggest that it is increasing. In its briefing document on the statistics, the Miscarriage Association says that,

"The most conservative estimate is that 1 in 5 pregnancies ends in miscarriage, usually in the first trimester. . . , but today the estimate is thought to be 1 in 4. The actual rate is probably higher than this, and nearer 1 in 3 (if not 2 in 5) and this takes no account of those miscarriages which go unreported as well as those taking place before the woman knows she is pregnant."

(Atik 1994)

In 1992 she estimated the number of miscarriages as "at least 200,000, probably nearer 300,000 and quite possibly up to 400,000."

Although there is disagreement over the number of Caesarean operations carried out in the UK, there is no dispute that the numbers have increased and are likely to be higher. (Stuttaford 1994c) There has also been concern about the number of deaths among women in childbirth, with critics showing that some hospitals are failing to follow safety measures intended to pinpoint early indications of problems. (Rogers 1994, Dept. Health 1994)

Those problem pregnancies which end in the baby's death are categorised according to the time of death. The Office of Population Censuses and Surveys (OPCS) draws the following distinctions:

28 complete weeks of gestation to birth – stillbirth
Stillbirths and deaths in the first week of life – perinatal death
Birth to 28 days – neonatal death
Death when over 28 days but under one year of age – postnatal death

Overall the trend has been downward in all the categories. For example, in 1980 the perinatal death rate was 13.3 per 1,000 total births. (England and Wales) (OPCS 1984) In 1991 it was 8 per thousand. (OPCS 1991a) The figures on congenital malformations are difficult to assess fully as many malformed fetuses are aborted. Thus although the number seems lower than twenty years ago, one has to remember that the abortion rate has risen. Taking the figures for spina bifida, for example, the rate has fallen from 15.3 in 1977 to 4.0 in 1986 and 1.5 in 1991 per 10,000 live births. However, in a South Australian study, it was found that the incidence of spina bifida had shown a decrease correlated to a rise in the number of therapeutic abortions. (Chan 1993) It is possible that a similar situation prevails here, though with the advice now given on folate supplementation (see Vitamins) one would expect a genuine fall in the incidence. Congenital malformations as a whole have decreased from 215.8 in 1977 to 197.1 in 1986 to 101.5 in 1991 per 10,000 per live births. But there were still 7,127 babies born with congenital malformations, including 6,889 live births. (OPCS 1991b) Ear malformations and cardiovascular problems have slightly increased over the last ten years. (OPCS 1987)

Sperm counts in a number of studies across the world would seem to be falling. One global study shows a drop of 50 percent. (Carlsen 1992)

In the USA the situation is also disappointing. Dr Harold Buttram compiled a list of facts which made dismal reading. Low birth weight babies were 1 for every 15 births. Doctor and hospital costs for initial hospitalization of a low birth weight baby can range from $16,136 to $174, 278 compared to $2,923 for the birth of a normal weight baby. 11 percent of all American schoolchildren are learning disabled. Childhood asthma has increased by about 40 percent during the last ten years. Spina bifida is 1 per 1000 births and 5 per 100 for women who already have an affected child. (Buttram 1994)

The fact is that whichever way one looks at the figures, for either the USA or UK, they show a great deal of misery and suffering for those directly involved in each tragedy and an enormous financial loss to society. Yet the research shows that much, if not most of the suffering could be avoided. Doctors are in the fortunate position of being able to take direct action to prevent some of the tragedies, although they cannot do it alone. Much depends on government action on pollution and general health promotion policies.

There are three main sections to the book:

Section One
looks briefly at the statistics which show that problem pregnancies are still too high for complacency about the standards of health care in Britain, or the United States of America. It gives advice on setting up a prepregnancy/ preconception care clinic before giving in detail the FORESIGHT protocol which has proved so successful in helping couples achieve healthy babies. (Ward 1993)

Section Two
has a brief overview of the types of problems associated with poor pregnancy outcome and some discussion of the causes, either known or suspected.

Section Three
is an A – Z of specific topics selected for their relevance to preconception and pregnancy outcome. It presents the research and rationale behind the protocol in section one.

Also included throughout the book are charts related to research conducted on the Foresight approach. The following abbreviations apply to these charts:

NH – No History	fert – no obvious infertility
Inf – infertile	low sp – low sperm count
Mis – miscarriage	p mot – poor motility
THTE – therapeutic termination	mal s – malformed sperm
STIL – stillbirth	SFD – small for date/low birthweight
MAL – malformation	

The Appendices are included for photocopying as required, for patients. An address list (Appendix one) is also included for you to obtain further information on some of the topics. The books, booklets, posters, leaflets and questionnaires can be purchased from FORESIGHT.

If you wish to be kept informed of developments in the field of preconception care you may wish to join FORESIGHT, a British charity (non-profit making organisation) concerned with the promotion of preconception care. Membership will entitle you to a newsletter three times a year giving information of the latest research. Details are available from:

FORESIGHT
28 The Paddock
Godalming
Surrey GU7 1XD
England
Telephone 01483 427839 9.30am–6 pm (UK times please)
Fax 01483 427668

2 Setting up a Clinic

Whether a preconception care service is to be offered by a medical practice within its existing clinics or as a separate one, certain aspects must be provided if it is to be successful. This will apply whether or not the service is being conducted within an existing health service, such as the National Health Service in the UK, or privately.

These essentials include:

1 Staff training
A general survey of the literature about preconception suggests that there are many factors a preconception practitioner needs to consider. These include nutrition, genito-urinary infections, mineral melabolism, allergy, intestinal infestation, environmental toxins and natural family planning methods. FORESIGHT (UK) runs regular seminars and other organisations such as the British Society for Nutritional Medicine also hold regular conferences. (See Appendix one)

2 Laboratory services
Access is needed to good laboratory services which can analyse blood, stool and urine samples as appropriate. In the UK hair mineral analysis is not yet (1995) available on the National Health Service. Doctors may consider using the research facilities of the University of Surrey. This is possible through FORESIGHT. The University cannot deal directly with individuals. Please contact FORESIGHT for details.
Sweat analysis is also useful but this is only available through Biolab, London and must be done in person there. Biolab will also handle hair and blood samples. (See Appendix one)

3 Genito-urinary clinic

Access is also needed to a good genito-urinary clinic, if possible where colposcopy examination is available.

Organising the preconception clinic

Preconception care is necessarily time-consuming, although it may save time in the long run. Patients may not present with problems subsequently. The initial consultation needs at least one hour because it is so thorough. However, much of the advice and care on nutrition, contraception, avoidance of toxic substances including alcohol and tobacco, infections and infestations can be given by nursing staff after specific training. Ideally, advice on diet and supplements should be given by a nutritionist/dietician, but those who have the necessary knowledge are rare in doctors' practices so another member of the team may need training.

Dr Marilyn Glenville has suggested a number of ways to organise the clinic. (Glenville Undated) There could be just one doctor involved, or health visitors, practice nurses or midwives may choose to organise the clinic, using the services of the doctor for medical examinations and tests. Patients may be seen alone, in couples, or in groups, depending on the individual circumstances and what the practice can manage.

An introductory letter for referring patients is useful. (See Appendix five) It may help to encourage patients if they know what to expect at the first consultation. It may also be helpful if the patient has prepared some information – FORESIGHT has a useful questionnaire. (See Appendix six) It is helpful to have certain other information available to give/lend to patients including:

a List of local organic food producers or shops. The doctor may be able to come to a local arrangement with some of them to supply fliers or a poster.

b A supply of literature for patients, maybe a small library of books as contained in the recommended reading list. (See Appendix two) As a minimum one could consider:

Planning for a Healthy Baby;
The FORESIGHT Wholefood Cookbook;
The FORESIGHT Video *Preparing for the Healthy Baby;*
Preparing for Pregnancy;
Find Out;
The Adverse Effects of Tobacco Smoking on Reproduction;
The Adverse Effects of Alcohol on Reproduction;
The Effects of Food Additives on Health,
The Adverse Effects of Lead,
The Adverse Effects of Genitourinary Infections with Particular Reference to

Fertility in Preconception Care;
The Adverse effects of Zinc Deficiency.

c Details of local branches of organisations such as National Childbirth Trust, Soil Association, FORESIGHT, Fertility Trust (for Natural Family Planning) Addresses can be found in Appendix one.

Who should be the target?

Glenville has identified a number of couples and women who would benefit from the preconception programme advocated in this book.
They include:

1 Normal healthy, fertile couples who want to do the best for their babies.

2 Couples who have general infertility with or without known cause, including problems with sperm count, motility, anovulation, etc.

3 Couples with single or recurrent spontaneous abortions.

4 Couples with a previous history of malformation, prematurity, low birth weight, stillbirth or sudden infant death syndrome.

5 Couples seeking preconception advice for IVF, GIFT and IUI. Couples preparing for a healthy baby and also hoping to increase the chances of conception where the success rate is already low (25% at best for IVF).

6 Older couples including women over 40 years, especially for help in preventing Down's syndrome. (Glenville Undated)

7 Couples where one of the partners has a malformation or chronic health problems, eg. epilepsy, multiple sclerosis, diabetes, eczema, myalgic encephalomyelitis, asthma, migraine.

3 Preconception Medical Check
– The FORESIGHT Way

The aim of the preconception care program is to help BOTH parents attain optimum health before their child is conceived. In this way one can optimise the chance of a the baby being born healthy. The preconception medical check is the first stage in the programme; this has been compiled from the experience of FORESIGHT UK doctors and FORESIGHT USA.

The timing of intervention

Present knowledge shows that the best time to start preconception care would be during the parent's embryonic and fetal stages, since that is when the physical structure is developed and the ova are formed in the ovaries. If, for example, a mother smokes during pregnancy, research has indicated that her subsequent daughter may give birth to a child who is not of optimum health. (Hawkes 1994d) Professor David Barker has shown that the mother's nutrition in early pregnancy may be linked with heart disease in her offspring in their later life. (Barker 1990) (See Nutrition)

Realistically, though, most people start their planning much later, so this information is only of use in reinforcing that their planning and work at this stage will benefit not only their child, but possibly any subsequent grandchild. It can also be stressed that there is considerable research to suggest that even short-term planning is beneficial in all but a very few cases.

In a biological sense the life process (and the developmental hazards) begin about 100 days before conception, when both the male and female germ cells (sperm and ova) commence their maturation process. During these processes, both ova and sperm are extremely vulnerable to nutritional deficiencies, toxins and radiation. One of the problems of famine has been mentioned above. Problems may occur even for four months or so after the food shortage has finished. Women who had taken medicinal drugs in the three weeks preceding conception have been found to have a higher risk of chromosomal aberrations. Radiation affecting the male germ cells has been linked with later congenital defects. It is also known that if the female germ cells in animals are irradiated on the day before conception there is a much greater incidence of chromosomal abnormalities. (Wynn 1986. Wynn 1981)

The International Commission for the Protection against Environmental Mutagens and Carcinogens (ICPEMC) has recommended that the male needs three months to recover from exposure to mutagens, such as radiation. However, two leading researchers, Arthur and Margaret Wynn, disagree with this, concluding after a review of all the literature that there should be a minimum of four months:

> "The Information from the Dutch Hunger Winter suggests that the whole legacy of disease, like childhood cancer and congenital malformations, that may have been caused by new mutations, originated mainly during the four months and particularly during the four weeks before conception."   (Wynn 1986)

RECOMMENDATION: FORESIGHT recommends preconception care planning starts six months before a planned conception. This enables time for tests to be completed and the results to be obtained. Obviously this time may need to be increased subject to the doctor's medical check. See typical presenting problems in Tables 1 and 2; data from University of Surrey study 1993.

The initial consultation

The following is a guide to the initial consultation. Before it occurs the doctor may wish to send out an introductory letter. (See Appendix five)

Co-operation with the Couple's Medical/General Practitioner: At the beginning of the programme the co-operation of the couple's own doctor should be sought. All records should be available to him/her.

Medical History
Much of the background for this can be obtained by asking both partners to complete a detailed questionnaire, an example of which is given in Appendix six. It is important to set aside enough time for discussion of the many relevant matters, including:
Life-style;
Work;
Hobbies;

Table 1 : Percentage (%) of Female Cases with no History or with Types of Previous Reproductive Problems – based on 367 women
(Ward 1993)

Reproductive problems	%	Specific details
No history	41	
Infertility	37	Period: 11% <1yr, 36% < 2yr, 33% > 5yr, 7% > 10yr
Miscarriage	38	Number: 63% only 1, 14% only 2, 16% only 3, 3% only 4 or 5
Therapeutic abortions	11	Number 89% only 1, 11% only 2
Stillbirths	3	
SIDS	1	
Small-for-date/low birthweight (<2300g)	15	11% small-for-date
Malformations	2	Spina bifida

Table 2 : Medical History of 367 couples (Ward 1993)

Condition	%	Condition	%
Acne	8	Griping after meals	4
Anorexia	1	Grooved tongue	3
Asthma	5	Hair loss	8
Back pain	32	Halitosis (bad breath)	14
Bleeding gums	26	Headaches/migraines	39
Bloated after meals	30	High blood pressure	<1
Blood shot eyes		High raised palate	<1
Body odour (severe)	<1	Hives	3
Bowel cramps	18	Hostility (no cause)	6
Brittle nails	20	Hyperactivity	3
Bruising (no cause)	6	Insomnia	11
Burning feet	5	Irritable bowel	13
Catarrh	29	Joint pain	16
Coeliac disease	<1	Kidney disorders	1
Cold feet	48	Memory loss	9
Cold hands	30	Mouth ulcers	19
Colitus	3	Multiple sclerosis	1
Constipation	28	Nervousness	15
Cystitus	9	Palpitations	9
Dandruff	25	Panic attacks	6
Dental decay	15	R Arthritis	1
Depression	21	Sciatica/lumbago	6
Diarrhoea	14	Sensitivity to noise	13
Dizzy spells	10	Stretch marks	23
Dyslexia	1	Sweating (heavy)	3
Ear infections	5	Tinnitus	7
Eczema	9	Urticaria	6
Enlarged glands	5	Varicose veins	15
Epilepsy	<1	Weight problems (low)	2
Fatigue/lethargy	41	(high)	15
Urinating frequently	17	White spot on nails	27

Family medical histories, ideally as far back as grandparents. This should include genetic problems in the family or ethnic background; (Reading 1984)
Diet, including any food allergies/intolerances;
Chemical exposures in the home or workplace;
Drug taking, including the contraceptive pill and self-prescribed medication;
Prescribed medication;
Smoking pattern;
Alcohol intake;
Personal medical history, especially previous pregnancies, diabetes, eczema, asthma, migraine, epilepsy, heart conditions, and infections; (See Appendix six)
Stress factors.

The following tests should be considered in the light of the medical history.

Blood Pressure
High blood pressure will often respond to dietary intervention.

Blood examination
Routine blood tests recommended include a complete blood count with white and red blood cells. Where indicated by the history, blood chemistries including blood sugar, electrolytes, kidney and liver function tests, uric acid, cholesterol and its fractions, a thyroid profile: red blood cell mineral analysis, serum vitamin profile, rubella antibodies and serology for syphilis. Where necessary tests can also be done for conditions such as sickle cell disease and thalassaemia, an eosinophil count to indicate an active allergy.

Basal Temperature
This is thought to be a reliable way of testing thyroid function. If the thyroid is underactive there will be insufficient sex hormone output and ovulation may not take place. (Barnes 1976) Basal temperature is also used to determine whether or not ovulation is happening. Special thermometers are available and may be easier to use. The test involves placing a thermometer under the arm for ten minutes every morning immediately on waking for two menstrual cycles. If the temperature is low for the whole of the cycle, a thyroid function test should be considered. Kelp, B_1 and manganese will be helpful with thyroid function. (Davies 1954, Pfeiffer 1978)

Semen samples
An up-to-date semen sample should be examined where there is any reason to suspect that the sperm could be abnormal, which may happen where there is a recent history of chronic ill health, coeliac condition, alcoholism, heavy drug

use, including smoking, debilitating illness and/or surgery. A semen sample should also be taken where a couple has been trying to start a baby for some time without success, or where the female has become pregnant and had a miscarriage or stillbirth or where the male has fathered a child who has suffered a congenital malformation. In cases of infertility semen should be cultured for infection also.

Genito-urinary examination
The doctor will need to make a full genito-urinary examination, especially for infection. Doctors who specialise in preconception clinics are finding such a high level of infection among their patients, that they consider a screening for genito-urinary infections should form part of any preconception medical check. (See Adverse conditions) It may be necessary to do a prostatic massage and to culture the prostatic secretions. Many genito-urinary infections are asymptomatic until the hormonal changes of early pregnancy stimulate the organisms to reproduce.

Both partners should be checked for the following:

Gonorrhoea	Anaerobic bacteria	Gardnerella
B. Strep	Staph. Aureas.	Candida
Chlamydia	Heam. Influenza	Ureaplasmas
Heam. Strep.	Mycoplasmas	Strep Millerii
Enterococcus	E. coli	Herpes
Klebsiella		

Non STDs: Toxoplasmosis Cytomegalovirus Rubella immunity
One FORESIGHT clinician found 69% of patients positive for one or more infections. (Nevison 1993)

Urine analysis
This should be done to check for protein and sugar and, if necessary, kidney infection.

Stool samples
Where indicated by a history of irritable bowel syndrome, or where the hair mineral analysis shows very low levels of minerals, a stool sample should be taken to check for malabsorption and/or worm and giardia or other intestinal infestations. Anything which can interfere with the ingestion of nutrients can have serious repercussions for fertility and pregnancy outcome.

Dental health
The patients should be advised to have a dental check-up done and to ensure that all treatment is completed at least four months before conception. Their

dentist should be asked not to use amalgam fillings as these contain mercury. The patient should be informed that cavities or gum infections are less likely to develop on an adequate diet.

Drinking water samples

If the hair mineral analysis shows high levels of copper, lead, cadmium, mercury and/or aluminum the patients should be advised to have their drinking water analysed to check that the levels are within the World Health Organisation's limits. If levels are high the matter should be referred to the relevant authority. In the UK this is the local Environmental Health Officer. In the USA it can be checked by National Testing Laboratories Inc.

The patient should be advised to use a water filter, first checking a sample after filtration. If the sample is also high then bottled water should be used. The patient should be warned to use the filter in accordance with the manufacturer's recommendations, or toxins could build up in it.

Allergy, malabsorption and/or intestinal infestation

This may include asthma, eczema, migraine, insomnia, depression, irritable bowel syndrome; coaliac disease or parasitic infestations such as giardia lamblia. With dietary manipulation, or antibiotic treatments, a lot of medication that is contraindicated in pregnancy may be avoided. Where parasites are eliminated the absorption of essential nutrients will be much improved. Where the history reveals a chronic problem likely to be incompatible with a healthy pregnancy, specialist help should be sought.

Sweat test

This is a test for mineral levels which is said to be a reliable indicator of magnesium and zinc status. Currently it is only available at Biolab, England,(See Appendix one) and the patient must visit the laboratory in person. It is especially useful where there is a doubt about zinc or magnesium status.

Hair mineral analysis

A sample of hair is taken from the scalp and is analysed using very sophisticated spectroscopy equipment, often down to 0.1 parts per million or less. Such detailed analysis is useful as some minerals are only found in hair in very small amounts, reflecting the small amounts found in the body.(Vitale 1975) However, even very small amounts can play a crucial part in maintaining health and reproductive competence.

Hair as a screening tool has a number of advantages over other tissues or fluids. (Laker 1982. Klevay 1978. Maugh 1978. Gordon 1980. Fletcher 1982) Samples can be taken easily, stored without elaborate arrangements and sent in an ordinary envelope. There is no risk of infection and it is inexpensive compared with many other tests. Urine only gives information about what the body is excreting, while blood can only show what is in it at the time the sample is taken. Moreover, since minerals in the blood are kept at near-optimum levels by a homeostatic mechanism, minor deficiencies are not always detectable at an early stage through blood samples. Many toxins, such as heavy metals, are passed out of the blood into other tissues. Thus, blood does not accurately reflect what is in the body stores. (Vitale 1975)

However, hair grows slowly and a properly taken sample can give a history of what has been passed into the hair follicle in the previous six to eight weeks. Moreover, hair contains high levels of many minerals, often 200 times greater than in the blood. Hair mineral analysis is a useful screening tool and, especially when done in combination with blood and sweat tests, gives a picture of what is happening in the body that is adequate for clinical purposes as a guide to mineral status.

Even used on its own it can still provide a good survey of what is happening in the body, if it is interpreted by an expert who knows what part each mineral plays in maintaining health. Indeed, there are over 1,500 citations in the scientific and medical literature confirming its usefulness. (Passwater 1983) The experts who use it continually are convinced that it is a valid medical test, but stress that it is only as good as the technician carrying out the analysis and the person interpreting the results.

NB *The oft-quoted study, 'Commercial Hair Analysis: Scam or Science?', purporting to prove it is unreliable was so poor it should never have been printed, let alone published in a major medical journal. (Barrett 1985) (The only point it proved was the inadequacy of peer review!)*

Dr Barrett, who conducted the study, claimed to have shown "that the reported levels of most minerals varied considerably between identical samples sent to the same laboratory". However, in an excellent critique, Dr Schoenthaler has pointed out that the study was poorly designed and statistically incorrect. (Schoenthaler 1986) For example, the researchers took the samples incorrectly without telling the laboratories, and ignored the fact that the laboratories derived their norms according to criteria that pertained to more stringent sampling methods. In a re-analysis of the data, Schoenthaler showed that there was a very high degree of reliablity (96 per cent) between five laboratories, and an average of 92 per cent between the "best" seven. In fact, when more meticulously examined, Barrett's data proved the opposite of what he was claiming!

It was therefore quite worrying that the Lancet should have used Barrett's work as the basis for an Editorial criticising the use of hair mineral analysis in preconception care. (Lancet 1985)

The Foresight experience and their research conducted with the University

of Surrey has shown that hair analysis is vitally important. (Ward 1993)
RECOMMENDATION: No preconception care examination is complete
without a hair mineral analysis, as mineral status is the most important factor
in ascertaining health before conception.

Nutrition

Couples may be given the *FORESIGHT Wholefood Diet* leaflet and the *FORESIGHT
Wholefood Cookbook*.The dangers from food additives must be explained.
FORESIGHT can provide a booklet *Find Out* and a summary by Tuula Tuormaa
The Adverse Effects of Food Additives on Health. Couples are advised to buy
organic foods whenever possible. FORESIGHT branch secretaries can give a list
of local organic suppliers.

Common social poisons

Both partners are fully informed of the dangers of smoking, alcohol and street
drugs to the health and development of sperm and ova and to the future of the
fetus. Both partners are advised to abstain for at least four months prior to
conception. This can be reinforced by the summaries of Tuula Tuormaa, *The
Adverse Effects of Tobacco Smoking on Reproduction* and *The Adverse Effects
of Alcohol on Reproduction.*

Contraception and Family Planning

Since it is important that the couple avoids pregnancy until their health is
optimum, appropriate family planning advice is essential. The doctor will
need to ascertain what methods of contraception have been used in the past. If
these have included the contraceptive pill, any other hormonal methods, or
any intra-uterine device, screening for mineral status and infections become
even more important. Hormonal contraceptive methods will give rise to mineral
imbalances and both hormonal and IUD methods encourage infections. It is
therefore essential that patients are advised to avoid these methods.

Recommended Contraception Methods include Natural Family
Planning and barrier methods.

Natural Family Planning (NFP) is recommended by FORESIGHT either
with abstention or with the use of a barrier method on fertile days. However,
it is recognised that some couples may prefer to use a barrier method all the
time, though this is generally unnecessary. An advantage of NFP is that it
teaches fertility awareness and this can be important when a couple have
fertility problems. They can use both temperature charts and mucus observation
for accuracy.

Since NFP is not always understood a brief overview is given in the
A-Z guide in this book. NFP needs to be taught properly. Addresses where
teachers may be obtained are in Appendix one. (The clinic may wish to consider

training a nurse in the practice to teach it.) Barrier methods are also included in the A-Z. A video on NFP is available from the Fertility Trust. (See Appendix one)

The Follow-up Consultation

When the various test results are known, the couple should be seen to discuss the results and be advised on treatment. Advice needs to include:

Counselling on diet, nutritional supplements, cleansing programmes and filtering the water;

Obtaining organic food and the avoidance of food additives;

The avoidance of toxins and how to cleanse the body of those already known to be present;

Avoidance of smoking, alcohol and drugs;

Treatment of chronic and genitourinary diseases and/or infestations;

Management of allergies;

Emotional support;

Natural family planning and advice on barriers;

Genetic counselling, if necessary;

Filtering the drinking and cooking water.

The A-Z pages gives full guidance about these topics.

Following the full programme, the pregnancy can be started with a normal, strong sperm and ova, the embryo can implant in a healthy uterus and can develop in optimum conditions. There will be no danger from nutritional deficiency, or damage from heavy metals or other toxins or viral and/or bacterial disease.

FORESIGHT has found that under these conditions it is possible to have uncomplicated pregnancies resulting in strong healthy and perfectly formed babies.

SECTION TWO

INFERTILITY AND
PROBLEM PREGNANCY OUTCOMES

In this section the focus is initially on infertility and then on the most common problem pregnancy outcomes. Not all may be thought to be associated with pregnancy – cardiovascular disease at age 50 years, for example. However, research is showing that the prepregnancy and pregnancy periods may affect the health, mental and physical, of future children at any stage of their lives.

Infertility

Infertility is thought to be present when a couple fail to start a pregnancy within a year or so of trying. Winston recommends seeking advice after eighteen months. (Winston 1986) The incidence of infertility is not known, though there have been a number of studies which suggest figures of about one in ten or one in eight, with one in six couples seeking help with a first or subsequent pregnancy. (Winston 1986, Varma 1987, Hall 1988) Authorities differ on how often the male or female is responsible, with assessments of the male contribution as between 30 and 50 per cent, depending on who is quoted. (Winston 1986, Onwudiegwu 1993)

There are many causes, and the FORESIGHT approach will not relieve infertility in every situation, though research has shown that it can help in a large number of cases because it tackles many of the factors which lead to problems of conception, especially biochemical imbalances and disease. The recent research study showed an 86 per cent success rate among couples who had followed the FORESIGHT programme. (Ward 1995)

In the woman there may be problems associated with:
1 Ovulation
The endocrine system may not be working properly to release the necessary hormones. Disease, severe nutritional disturbances, allergies, malabsorption, significant weight loss, strenuous physical activity, stress, exposure to chemical and physical agents, such as the pill or radiation, can also interfere with ovulation.

Where a failure to ovulate is suspected it is suggested that the FORESIGHT protocol is followed before the usual investigations outlined by Winston such as blood progesterone and prolactin measurements, hormone tests, ultrasound, endometrial biopsy and laparoscopy. Winston claims that, "For most problems with ovulation, the treatment is astonishingly effective," referring to drug treatments. (Winston 1986) Treatment with the drugs he outlines is not recommended as the first option by FORESIGHT as the drugs compromise nutritional status and often have serious side effects. There has been concern that women have been given fertility drugs without full investigation of their medical problems. (Pallot 1990) (See Drugs)

2 Structural faults
These may be congenital, with perhaps a lack of organs, or faulty organs. There may be blocked or twisted Fallopian tubes. The FORESIGHT protocol includes investigation of a number of factors which may be causing blockages, including genito-urinary infections, zinc deficiency or allergic oedema of the tissue of the tube, which has also been linked to a thickening of the fallopian secretions.

The tissue of the tube
When the causes are eliminated through nutritional and cleansing programmes, and where appropriate antibiotic treatments to eliminate infections have been given, the tubes sometimes clear to allow conception. Often, however, the tubes will have suffered physical damage such as scarring and adhesions and pregnancy through normal sexual intercourse is not possible. (See Assisted Pregnancy)
       Recent research has suggested that sperm need the assistance of muscle contractions in the womb if they are to reach the Fallopian tubes. The researcher said, "women who have difficulty conceiving with no obvious cause may have abnormalities in the direction, frequency or intensity of contractions. Their best chance is to pick the time of ovulation when the waves are likely to be at their most helpful." (Hawkes 1994a) The contractions are also encouraged by prostaglandins in the seminal fluid, so it would seem that the man should be encouraged to include essential fatty acids in his diet as these are needed in the production of prostaglandins. (Harrison 1990) The environment in the vagina, uterus and tubes may not be healthy enough to support the sperm through its journey. The uterus lining may not be healthy enough for implantation. There is some debate about problems with cervical mucus although Winston estimates that about 5 per cent of female infertility may be due to problems related to the mucus. (Winston 1986). The FORESIGHT experience has shown nutritional intervention to be successful in almost all cases.

3 Medical conditions
including, for example, endometriosis, polyps, and/or fibroids, or pelvic

inflammatory disease can affect fertility and sometimes pregnancy outcome. Genitourinary infection must be treated in both partners and rechecked.

4 Age
decreases fertility, though research suggests that under ideal conditions the effect of age on the chance of achieving a successful pregnancy may be less than previous studies supposed. (West 1987) The FORESIGHT experience has shown that women in their early 40s can have successful pregnancy outcomes with the correct preparation.

5 The egg
may not be healthy and may be incapable of developing after fertilisation. Alternatively, it may develop but produce abnormalities. It may also implant incorrectly to produce an ectopic pregnancy. This is particularly likely where tubes are partially blocked due to infection. The full FORESIGHT programme will nourish the ova and treat lingering infections.

6 If the egg is implanted, the woman may not be healthy enough to maintain the pregnancy, perhaps because of poor nutritional status, an over-high level of copper, (Vallee 1965) infections, allergic illness or the presence of toxins. Alternatively she may maintain her pregnancy, but have a premature birth or poor outcome. Zinc and/or magnesium deficiency need to be pre-empted.

7 Previous sterilisation may be a factor and reversal is not always successful.

In the man the main reasons for fertility problems include:
1 Absence of live sperm in the semen
This can arise because of structural problems, such as blocked or twisted seminal tubes, or no tubes at all. The endocrine system may not be working properly to stimulate the production of sperm. An injury or birth defect, such as an undescended testicle which has atrophied, may also be the cause.

2 Low sperm count
Winston suggests that this accounts for over 90 per cent of male problems. (Winston 1986) Generally speaking it is reckoned that a man has a low sperm count if he has less than 20 million sperm in a millilitre of semen. There have been a number of reports that male sperm counts have declined over the last few decades. One researcher has shown that 23 per cent of male students at Florida State University have sperm counts that are functionally sterile, that is lower than 20 million sperm per millilitre of semen, a result similar to the 20 per cent in other studies. This compares with 0.5 per cent in 1938. (Dougherty 1980) Another report mentions a decline of 50 per cent over the

last 30 years. (Carlsen 1992, Laurance 1992, Gill 1992) However, researchers in Edinburgh do not accept the evidence for falling sperm counts. (Irvine, 1994)

Reasons for low sperm count include:

a Nutritional imbalances. Vitamin E, Zinc, Vitamin B12 and many other nutrients are needed for healthy sperm.

b Chemicals in the home and workplace. (Taskinen 1989, Robaire 1993).

c Occupation, especially long-distance lorry-drivers, pilots, workers who are exposed to considerable vibrations, or any job which is very tiring and/or stressful.

d High levels of toxic metals such as lead or cadmium.

e Over heating of the testicle by tight clothing.

f Medical conditions such as varicocele, or abnormal blood vessels around the testes.

g Drugs, including those used in therapy for infertility or low sperm count itself. Tobacco and alcohol can be factors, as is marijuana. (Wynn 1985) Winston lists the following as possibly causal:

> "Antidepressants. . . Antimalarial drugs. . .
> Antihypertensives. . . Sulphasalazine. . . Cytotoxic drugs. . .
> Furandantin. . . Corticosteroids (this is not proven, but they may
> affect some men)."
>
> (Winston 1986)

h Infections.

i Hormonal problems which interfere with sperm production.

j Excessive exercise.

3 Impaired sperm function, unhealthy sperm

The sperm may have poor motility and fail to reach the egg. If there is a lack of zinc the sperm may fail to penetrate the egg. Infection with chlamydia will also affect sperm function as will social drugs, such as smoking and alcohol, and some medicinal drugs.

4 Antibodies

Sometimes the man has antibodies to his own sperm which may even prevent the sperm from being released at all.

5 Physical problems which may, for example, cause difficulty with sexual intercourse, or may mean the sperm are not ejaculated into the vagina, as in

the case of hypospadias or retrograde ejaculation. The absence of organs such as the vas deferens or testes are rare problems. Injury to the male sex organs can cause difficulties. Sometimes chemicals can cause damage to the testes, as in the case of phthalates. (Nuttall 1994a)

6 There may have been a previous vasectomy and the blood may make antibodies to the sperm. (See also Appendix six)

Caesarean births

Although the outcome of a caesarean birth may be eventually a healthy child, this is not the case at the time of the birth, since both baby and mother will have been exposed to some drug(s). Obviously caesarean sections are sometimes essential for the safety of the mother and/or baby.

However, there is now rising concern over the numbers of such sections being carried out, although there is a dispute over the actual rise. The Royal College of Obstetricians and Gynaecologists report an increase from 10 percent in 1988 to 14.5 percent in 1992 to 15.3 percent in 1993, while another researcher says the increase is 2.4 percent on average between 1992 and 1993. (Friend 1994, Francombe 1994) The rate is four times higher than twenty years ago. In the US the rate is higher still.

A further worry is the widely differing rates between maternity units. A National Child Birth study shows a range from 9 percent to 22 percent. (Laurance 1994) It is difficult to assess reasons for the increase, though some of it is almost certainly due to better technology and procedures which enable difficult vaginal deliveries which may be potentially damaging to mother and/ or baby to be avoided.

Whatever the actual figures, a caesarean section should be regarded as a problem pregnancy outcome and prepregnancy preparation should aim to minimise its use. The FORESIGHT programme should ensure the mother enters labour replete in zinc, copper, magnesium and B complex vitamins and all other necessary nutrients. This means a vigorous labour, with strong contractions and less likelihood of "labour fade". Caesareans on account of prolonged labour are thus less likely.

Many caesareans are forced on mother and practitioner, however, by narrow pelvic development in the mother leading to disproportion. It is hoped that the new generation of girls born to mothers who have followed the FORESIGHT programme with its adequate diet will have more propitious skeletal development.

The research of Dr Weston Price and Dr Francis Pottenger show that there is reason to believe that with this nutritional intervention future generations can escape the disadvantage of poor skeletal structure. (Pottenger 1983, Price 1945)

Chronic illness in babies

Unfortunately a number of babies will be born with chronic illness, sometimes infected by their mother. This can occur with a number of genito-urinary infections, the main one being chlamydia. (See Adverse conditions). Others may have heart defects or respiratory problems, which may be associated with infections or may be the result of poor prenatal and antenatal care. (See Drugs, Minerals, Nutrition, Toxic Metals, Vitamins) Allergies can be very debilitating and often go undiagnosed for years. Where any child has chronic health problems it is advisable to check for genito-urinary infections, infestations, his/her nutritional status, and toxin levels.

Deaths in childbirth

In 1993 the number of women dying because of pregnancy and childbirth rose for the first time in fifteen years. A Department of Health report on confidential enquiries into maternal deaths in the UK between 1988 and 1990 found that in 49 per cent of the 238 maternal deaths there was evidence of sub-standard care. Hypertensive disorders were the leading cause of death at 18.6 per cent; of these 88 per cent received sub-standard care (Dept Health 1994). The charity, Action for Victims of Medical Accidents, has expressed concern about the number of deaths. The Association for Improvements in Maternity Services (Aims) has called for an investigation and is worried about the number of ruptured uterises. (Rogers 1994)

Lactation

There is now no dispute that "Breast is best". When the baby is born the first liquid from the breast is colostrum, which is rich in antibodies, essential fats and zinc. This is vital for the baby's immune system and is the reason why colostrum should always be the first substance ingested by the baby. Babies who are put on formula feeds from birth often develop allergies to cow's milk protein. (Eagle 1986) Human milk is also rich in antibodies, especially if the mother is healthy. Even though there have been reports that breast milk has high levels of pesticides and other toxins, they are also likely to be present in baby foods, unless they are prepared from organically grown foods. The incidence of toxins may be considerably reduced if the mother eats an organic diet.

Lactation problems can cause misery for mother and baby. The hungry baby will cry and fail to thrive at a time when his/her developing brain needs good nutrition. Too little milk may lead to supplementing with formula feeds which can only approximate human milk. Nipples of a mother who has nutritional deficiencies may be sore, making feeding difficult. These problems seem to occur less frequently in mothers who have followed and continue to follow the FORESIGHT progamme.

Low birth weight (See preterm babies)

Malformation/Chromosomal abnormality

Various animal and human research has shown that malformations can be caused and eradicated by manipulation of the diet. (Jennings 1970, Price Pottinger 1945, Underwood 1977, Hurley 1980, Smithells 1983, Prasad Oberleas and Caldwell 1970.,Vallee 1965) (See Chemicals, Hazards, Minerals, Nutrition, Radiation, Toxic Metals) It is now recognised that the chromosomal abnormality, Downs' syndrome, may be the responsibility of either the male or female. (Magenis 1977) Recent FORESIGHT research showed no malformations in a study of 327 couples who had completed their programme, though most had had previous problems in pregnancy, including 7 babies born with malformations. (Ward 1993)

Miscarriage

There are no reliable figures for the true incidence of miscarriage since where it occurs early in the pregnancy the woman may confuse it with a period. However, some say that one in four women who become pregnant will have one or more miscarriages. (Huisjes 1984) Among the causes that can be investigated after a miscarriage are:

Nutritional status: nutritional deficiencies and/or an excess of copper are linked with miscarriage.

Toxins: for example, lead, cadmium and/or aluminium levels and certain chemicals used in industrial processes. Drugs are also a problem, including social drugs such as alcohol and tobacco.

Radiation: this can be ionising or non-ionising.

Hormonal: an imbalance of hormones can trigger an abortion.

Physical factors: if the organs, such as the uterus, are misshapen, the woman may have difficulty in maintaining the pregnancy.

Infections: genito-urinary infections are often the cause.

Diseases: the risks of German measles are well-known but other conditions may also present problems, especially if there is fever.

Poor sperm quality: See Appendix six on male infertility leaflet.

Chromosomal factors: at least 30 per cent of aborted fetuses show chromosomal defects. (Winston 1986) Problems may be greater where both parents have chromosomal defects which the fetus inherits. However, Jennings' work has shown that given the right nutrients before and during pregnancy some chromosomal defects can be avoided. (Jennings 1970)

Immunological factors: these are still the subject of investigation but there is some suggestion that miscarriage may occur where there is an immunological incompatability between prospective parents. (Winston 1986)

The FORESIGHT experience suggests that the rate of miscarriage can be

Table 3 : Hair Zinc Concentration and Smoking Activity

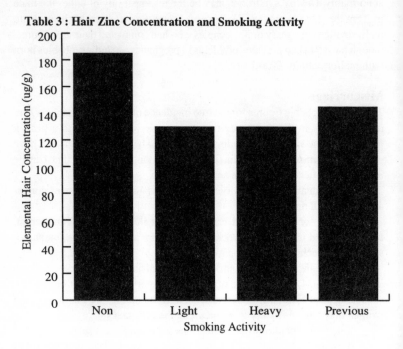

**Table 4 : Influence of Previous Reproductive Problems on Foresight
Pregnancy Outcome* (birthweight and gestational age)**
(367 couples, Ward 1993)

Previous history	Sex*(%)		Mean birthweight (g)	Mean gest. age (wks)
	Male	Female		
No history	37	63	3384	39
Infertility	44	56	3166	38
Miscarriage	52	48	3138	38
Therapeutic Therm.	36	64	3143	38
Stillbirths	0	100	3017	38
Small-for-dates (low-for-weight)	50	50	3060	38
Malformations	33	67	2887	37

*expressed as a percentage of pregnancy outcome for that group

dramatically reduced if their programme is fully followed by both partners. In a recent research study, conducted by the University of Surrey on the progress of 367 couples, there was a previous miscarriage rate of 83 per cent among the 59 per cent who had had a previous problem pregnancy. By the end of the study 96 per cent of couples in the full study had given birth, without any problems during the pregnancy. (Ward 1993)

Women who tend to have repeat miscarriages are more likely to have chromosomally normal aborted fetuses, so it seems likely that the fault lies in the mother's ability to carry the fetus, thus demonstrating the importance of her health. It has been questioned if a slow-down in the synthesis of DNA is a factor in early miscarriage, since a deficiency of many nutrients can slow it down, as well as causing chromosomal damage. (Bell 1975) This emphasises, yet again, that optimum nutrition is crucial.

At least one study has shown that a miscarriage occurring in the second trimester of pregnancy, especially at 19 -22 weeks, is associated with a higher risk of problems in the second pregnancy. Out of 95 women studied, 5 per cent had stillbirths and 6 per cent had neonatal deaths. For those who had previously miscarried between 19 and 22 weeks, 62 per cent of the births took place before the due date. (Goldenburg 1993) See also table 4. (Ward 1995)

Neo-natal deaths

The causes of neo-natal deaths are many. Sometimes such death may follow a difficult labour or birth accident. Many of the mothers seem to have suffered pre-eclamptic toxaemia, and the baby has been brought on too early to sustain life. Some babies may be born with a malformation that is incompatible with life.

The FORESIGHT programme seems to have been helpful with mothers who have had threatened pre-eclamptic toxaemia or even high blood pressure with previous pregnancies. Correcting the zinc levels and cleansing toxins, especially cadmium, seem to be important factors. Eliminating allergies and giving large doses of Vitamin C seem to help. Vitamin C may also help to reduce the level of pesticides, which are known to interfere with the metabolism of choline, an essential vitamin for liver function. Clearing up genito-urinary infections which might also affect kidney function may also be a factor.

Post partum depression

Post partum depression always has serious consequences for the family: the mother does not get the pleasure from her baby that is her right: the baby does not get the benefit of a healthy mother, which may lead to feeding problems and developmental problems: the father and any other children also suffer.

The situation usually need not arise. Depression is usually organic, allergic/biochemical in origin and responds to investigations as a physical disorder. When the mother has given birth she will have a high copper level, since copper is naturally raised at this time. Her zinc level will be low and, unlike animals, the human mother does not usually eat the placenta, the richest source of zinc known. Giving birth may cause abrasions, further lowering zinc levels as zinc is required for healing tissue. If she is zinc deficient , her milk will probably not contain the sufficient quantities for her baby to thrive and he/she may cry a lot. If the mother is manganese deficient, (and this is likely since people do not generally suffer from one deficient mineral alone) she may be confused and have difficulty organising herself at a time when she is having to make major adjustments. Zinc and manganese are factors in sugar metabolism, and deficiencies may lead to blood sugar swings, making the feelings of fatigue worse. In all cases of depression, vitamin and mineral supplements will prove helpful. If drugs are given they will cause nutritional imbalances, so the first approach should always be nutritional.

In one study it was found that 10 per cent of fathers suffered depression after the baby arrived home, with 5 per cent still depressed six months later. A state of Post-natal depression in men is confirmed by another report. (Stuttaford 1994b)

Depression is very rare in parents who have followed the FORESIGHT programme because their nutritional status is good throughout the pregnancy.

Pre-term and small-for-date babies

Preterm babies include those born early, before full term, who were previously known as premature births, and those babies who weigh less than 2500 grams (5lb 8oz) at birth. In some medical papers prematurity is still the word used for early births.

> "Between 6 and 8 percent of babies are born three weeks early, while 2 per cent are six weeks early and 1 per cent more than eight weeks premature. They are particularly at risk of developing respiratory syndrome and cerebral palsy, especially those born more than six weeks early."   (Tarnow-Mardi 1994)

Some writers give the causes for babies born with a short gestation period, (ie approximately 28 to 34 weeks after conception instead of 40 weeks), as:

Malnutrition;

Inadequate prenatal care;

Unfortunate socio-economic conditions;

Multiple pregnancies where the uterus walls cannot expand anymore;

Excessive smoking and/or alcohol;

Oxygen starvation;

Emotional disturbances (which probably affect nutritional status);

Drugs;

Age, especially where a young woman has a succession of babies;

First baby after 40 years of age;

Complications in pregnancy eg infections, toxaemia; (Annis 1978)

Heavy metal toxicity; (Ward 1987)

Births induced because of confusion over dates;

Low zinc/high copper imbalance; (Vallee 1965, Grant 1985)

Genito-urinary infection. (Grant 1985)

Other researchers highlight these factors and mention more. Prenatal malnutrition is undoubtedly a major damaging factor in low birth weight as famine studies have shown, though smoking more than 20 cigarettes a day doubles the risk. (Kamen 1981, Avery 1983) Deficiencies in essential fatty acids, Vitamin B1, calcium, copper, cobalt, magnesium and zinc are factors. (See vitamins and minerals) Other contributors include malformation of the uterus, fibroid tumours, high blood pressure, and genetic causes, such as maternal and paternal size, poor weight gain, poor obstetric history, stress and preterm labour. (Nance 1982)

Prolonged standing at work may also be a cause. (Naeye 1982) But it is probably inaccurate to regard many of these as reasons for low birth weight for the same reasons that many of the studies which quote demographic factors, such as socio-economic status, age, marital status and education may be misleading.

In the FORESIGHT experience these are not reasons in themselves: most can be linked with the mother's health status before and during pregnancy, especially the existence of infection, her nutritional status, her history of substance abuse and exposure to toxins such as heavy metals and drugs. Low socio-economic status may be the result of a poor educational status, and may mean low pay, with little money being spent on good food, assuming she is educated about the importance of healthy eating. Research shows smoking is more common in low income groups.

Premature babies may suffer from a range of physical, psychological and intellectual problems. (Lya den Ouden 1993) They have a wrinkled look and may be too weak to suck. Their brain may be too immature to control breathing or body temperature. They are prone to infection as their immune system is immature. (Lesser 1980) One study suggests that there is a need for long-term monitoring of babies born before 29 weeks of gestation as "the risk of impairment and disability increased with decreasing gestational age at birth ($p<0.003$)." (Johnson 1993)

Babies who weigh less than 2500 grams at birth are said to have a low birth weight. If they are under 1,500 grams they are of very low birth weight.

Table 5 : Birth Statistics for 327 Foresight Pregnancies (Ward 1993)

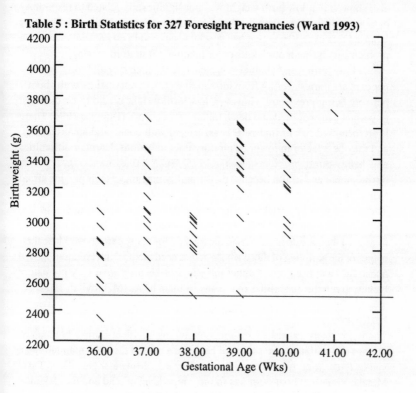

One study found that those with a birth weight between 2,000 – 2,500 grams will tend to have only slight problems which can be overcome with time. However, for those under 2,000 grams the outlook is poorer, and they are likely to have some type of developmental difficulty. (Cott 1985) Research by the National Perinatal Epidemiology Unit, Oxford, of 1,319 children found that the number of defects in vision was three times higher in those who had had low birth weights and the number suffering from ocular problems was proportional to the weight of the child if it was of low birth weight. The study also showed that low birth weight was not significantly related to respiratory or hearing difficulties, though other subtle changes were significant. Teachers reported that over 50 per cent had special needs and in 40 per cent there were problems with fine motor skills co-ordination. (Stuttaford 1994a)

Low birth weight babies represent 6 to 9 per cent of all births. About 2 per cent are born suffering from intrauterine growth retardation, with about 7 per cent being premature. However, low birth weight is said to be the most important cause of perinatal death (about 70 per cent). (Douglas 1984) There is an increased risk of illness. It is associated with congenital abnormalities, and may be a factor in lower respiratory tract infections, learning difficulties and behavioural problems.(Annis 1978) Such babies experience poorer development and health because their fragility may make their parents afraid to handle them and all babies need the stimulation of touch. (Churchill 1966) There may also be a risk of inferior intelligence-test achievements in late adolescence. (Seidman 1992) With better neonatal care, survival rates have improved, but this does not lessen the tragedy for many parents who lose their babies or the suffering of those whose babies need medical intervention. Indeed questions have been raised about the ethics of keeping alive very premature babies, given the disabilities that many of them have. (Marcovitch 1994)

Stillbirth

There are many causes of stillbirth, including accident during pregnancy, disease and malnutrition. Maternal health is a crucial factor in maintaining a viable fetus. (See Adverse conditions, Hazards, Minerals, Nutrition, Toxic Metals, Vitamins) FORESIGHT has found a high level of lead and /or cadmium in mothers suffering a previous stillbirth. (Ward 1993)

Subsequent health problems

There is now ample evidence to suggest that what happens in the womb can have repercussions for future health, much later in life than was thought earlier. Research on cardiovascular disease has shown that higher rates of deaths in areas where the babies had lower birth weights and were less likely to have been breastfed, suggested maternal health was important. Lower birth weight is associated with poorer maternal nutrition. The same team has started

Table 6: Foresight Male "Fertility" Status (367 males, Ward 1993)

"Fertility"	Percentage Reported
Sperm test	42
Antibodies	12
Low sperm count	30
Poor motility	35
Malformed sperm	5

In some cases a seminal fluid test was carried out by JSPS and MetPath (CLS). Data is provided on pH count, motility and abnormal forms in table below.

Table 7: Seminal Fluid Tests (JSPS and MetPath) (Ward 1993)

Conditions	Test and mean range		Ref value
Volume	5.0	2.4 – 6.8	–
pH	7.8	7.6 – 8.2	–
Count (million/ml)	121	45 – 350	50 –200
Motility			
Active (%)	60	42 – 85	
Sluggish (%)	20	5 – 35	
Non-motile (%)	30	20 – 48	
Abnormal forms (%)	<15	–	up to 40

"to identify the processes that link fetal infant growth with cardiovascular disease. A recent study of 449 men and women aged 50 years. . . showed that their current blood pressure and risk of hypertension were strongly related to their placental and birth weight. Pressures were highest when birth weight had been lower than expected from placental weight. Discordance between placental and birth weights may be interpreted as fetal growth failure. Its causes are unknown but maternal nutrition is an obvious suspect."   (Barker 1990, Prentice 1990)

An earlier study had linked adult high blood pressure and low birth weight. (Gennser 1988) Other conditions may also be linked with the maternal environment, including schizophrenia, obstructive lung disease, fetal alcohol syndrome, and diabetes. (Fine 1985, Noritoshi 1994). It would seem the role played by paternal smoking and alcohol, and by lead contamination of both parents is ripe for investigation in these types of study.

SECTION THREE

A–Z OF SPECIFIC TOPICS

A dverse Medical Conditions

This section contains information on diseases which are known to affect the fetus or child. Some of the conditions are well-known and only basic references are given. Others may not be so familiar so more detail about symptoms and treatment is included. A number of self-help and support groups are given in Appendix one. They are worth contacting as they tend to keep abreast of research, some of it not published in widely read journals.

Of particular importance in preconception screening are the checks for sexually transmitted diseases. The number of infected people continues to rise and most of the infections can have dire consequences for fertility, sterility, the fetus and the health of the sufferer. Some genito-urinary infections arise even between partners who are faithful to each other eg candidiasis. It should never be assumed there is no infection, since some of the conditions are asymptomatic. Often the conditions occur in combination and this multiplies the risk of damage. In one study, Mycoplasma hominis was found in 30 -50 per cent of vaginal cultures of sexually active women, with Ureaplasma urealyticum in 60 -80 per cent of cultures. (Gibbs 1987) Another study looked at the incidence of six infections in pregnant adolescents, aged 13 -17 years, all from poor socio-economic backgrounds and in their third trimester. The results showed that only five appeared to be free from all infections being considered, while 34 per cent had trichomonas, 38 per cent candidiasis, 70 per cent mycoplasma hominis, and 90 per cent Ureaplasma urealyticum. Chlamydia trachomatis was found in 37 per cent of 115 specimens. Gonorrhoea was originally present in 12 subjects in early pregnancy, but only in one in the third trimester. Three had evidence of genital herpes infection and three others evidence of papovirus infection. (Hardy 1984)

A survey of 109 patients attending a FORESIGHT clinic for preconception care confirmed the importance of screening. Of 32 men tested between November 1989 and May 1991, 15 had one or more infections. These included B Streptocci, Chlamydia trachomatis, Ureaplasma urealyticum, Staph Aureus, Candidiasis, Enteroccus, E coli, Klebsiella, Anaerobic bacteria, Haem influenza and Strep milleri. 77 women were tested, showing a total of 39 positive cervical swabs and 22 positive chlamydia antibodies. Infections identified included B Streptococci, ureaplasma, mycoplasma, anaerobic bacteria, candida, Gardnerella, E coli, Strep milleri, Staph/aureus. (Nevison, 1991)

In a study of 400 patients investigated immediately before abortion 28 per cent had anaerobic (bacterial) vaginosis, 24 per cent candidiasis, 8 per cent chlamydial infection, 0.75 per cent trichomonas infection and 0.25 per cent gonorrhoea. (Blackwell 1993)

While the immune system may cope with one mild infection, if there are multiple infections it is unlikely to be able to withstand such an onslaught. Comprehensive screening is essential, and where possible, this should always include the use of a colposcope, since it is a superior technique for at least one condition and it is thought to be a better one for others. (Schneider 1988, Sutton 1988) Preconception treatment for all infections is essential. This is especially crucial for any infection or cell abnormality on the cervix as the rise in hormones during pregnancy increases the problems. The extra hormone stimulation sometimes given to infertile women is particularly likely to cause a flare-up of cervical or pelvic infection. (Grant 1988) In many cases clearing up the infection may improve fertility of both partners.

AIDS –Acquired Immune Deficiency Syndrome

There is some uncertainty as to whether or not pregnancy will increase the risk of developing AIDS-related complex or the risk of the baby being infected in the womb in asymptomic women. Early studies suggest a risk. (Minkoff 1987) Other studies suggest no discernible effect. (Lindsay 1993)

Anaerobic Bacteria

There is some debate about whether or not the presence of anaerobic bacteria, including Gardnerella, in such abnormal amounts as to cause the condition bacterial vaginosis can cause an adverse outcome to pregnancy. Researchers at a leading UK hospital found that "late miscarriage and preterm delivery are associated with he presence of bacterial vaginosis in early pregnancy. This is independent of recognised risk factors such as previous preterm delivery". (Hay 1994)

Anorexia Nervosa – Bulimia

Both anorexia nervosa and bulimia may lead to infertility because of low levels of essential nutrients. Even if fertility is not a problem, the anorexic or bulimiac may put the fetus at risk because of these low levels. (See Nutrition, Minerals, Vitamins)

Some feminist writers believe that these conditions are attempts to cope in a world hostile to women. Others believe that eating is the only area in which the sufferer is able to exercise control over their life. Sufferers tend to be treated by psychiatrists though no psychiatric explanation has ever been proved. An approach which offers more hope is one including zinc supplementation, as first reported by Bryce-Smith and Simpson (1984). They cite a case of a patient making a full recovery from anorexia nervosa following zinc supplementation. It seems logical to assume that a disorder that is focused on eating will have some links with nutrition. Bryce-Smith and Hodgkinson have also suggested that "anorexia nervosa is basically a nutritional disorder resulting from greatly reduced food intake which may itself have social origins. This is combined, in susceptible people, with a probably inherited subnormal ability to utilise zinc." (Bryce-Smith 1986) Zinc is linked with the ability to smell and taste and if a person is deficient they are unlikely to enjoy their food, as they will not smell or taste it properly. It is therefore not so difficult to resist eating. The less food consumed the more nutritionally deficient the sufferer becomes and a vicious spiral ensues. He/she may suffer from diarrhoea, further compounding the problem. The muscles become soft and flabby and may be misidentified as "fat". (See Minerals) If there is no improvement in the condition after zinc supplementation the problem may be iron or magnesium deficiency. It is advisable to check mineral status carefully. Professor Bryce-Smith believes that about 15 per cent of patients do not improve, but there could be many reasons for this including failure to diagnose an oesophagal obstruction, infection or allergy.

There are a number of reasons why zinc supplementation should be the first choice of treatment:

1 Unlike all the psychiatric measures, there is no potential for harm. Of course, some counselling for patient and family may be beneficial, as there is always considerable anxiety, but it should be completely non-judgemental, merely supportive. Drugs and electro-convulsive therapy always have severe side effects, and behaviour therapy is inappropriate and cruel if the problem is physical.

2 It can be given, in drop form, even where the patient is uncooperative in treatment, since he/she does not need to know it is being given.

3 If a deficiency is the main problem, improvement in most cases will be rapid and the patient will not deteriorate too much before the treatment works.

4 It is easy to carry out the treatment at home.

5 It is cheap – often less than the cost of the fare to a medical centre!

Candidiasis (Thrush)

(This section has been written partly using notes prepared by Dr Harold Buttram.)

The yeast, Candida Albicans, occurs naturally in the human body, and in healthy people it causes no problems. It is well known as a cause of oral thrush and diaper rash (nappy rash) in babies. However, few issues in the medical field have been more controversial than that of candidiasis as a cause of systemic illness. This may have been because of difficulties of proof. Even those friendly to the concept have often questioned the value of tests to verify the condition. It is sometimes thought of as a phantom illness.

There is general agreement about the basic concepts surrounding candidiasis as a cause of systemic symptoms. When antibiotics are taken, they tend to kill off beneficial or "friendly" micro-organisms (bacteria) in the intestinal tract and other mucus membranes of the body, thereby allowing overgrowth of Candida, which is not affected by antibiotics. Overgrowth of the yeast in the intestinal tract results in increased production of toxins and allergenic substances which create bowel irritation and inflammation. Not only are these harmful substances absorbed into the blood stream, but the bowel itself may be impaired by inflammation, thereby leading to what is called "the leaky gut syndrome", with increased bowel permeability to incompletely digested food fragments and other antigenic substances. The immune system, increasingly burdened, at some point begins to decompensate. Other systemic symptoms ensue such as those of an irritable bowel, fatigue, and a worsening of allergies. (Crook 1983) In addition to antibiotics, prolonged use of the contraceptive pill or of cortisone derivatives are considered as risk factors for Candidiasis, as well as a high intake of sugar.

One authority has said that there was a doubling of new cases of genital candidiasis reported between 1971 and 1975. (Munday 1983) Such candidiasis may cause painful intercourse and possibly provide a hostile atmosphere for the sperm. Doctors at the University of Southern California have found that excessive antibiotics used to treat middle ear infections in childhood contributed to growth of yeast in the middle ear. It was only after treatment with an antifungal drug, ketoconazole, that the middle ears of the children improved. (Dohen 1990)

Work at Cornell University, New York, has demonstrated immune suppression from Candida albicans infections. In addition to creating an increased susceptibility to Candida re-infection, the resulting immunologic alterations may also be related to subsequent endocrinopathies and harmful auto antibody formation. (Witkin 1985) Case studies of patients with chronic fatigue syndrome reported by an Assistant Clinical Professor at the University of California at San Francisco showed that 80 per cent of them had a history of recurrent antibiotic treatment at some stage in their life.(Schmidt 1993)

Symptoms
The symptoms of chronic candidiasis are many. They may include allergies and sensitivity to food and/or chemicals, craving for carbohydrates and/or alcohol, alcohol intolerance and irritable bowel syndrome. Iron or zinc deficiency can affect nutritional status and may therefore compromise

reproductive outcomes (though, of course, any adverse state of health could do this!) (Davies 1987)

Diagnosis
Although it is now possible to test for gut infestation of Candida albicans, this is currently only possible at one laboratory in the UK. Diagnosis can be made by taking a medical history and also by swab. (Arrangements can be made through Biolab, London. See Appendix one)

Treatment
Most of the symptoms can be relieved with anti-fungal agents and nutritional therapy. Short courses of Vitamin A, which protects the mucus membranes, have been found to be helpful. The dose is a maximum of 21,000 IUs for three to four days, reducing to 7,000 IUs. This should be reduced to 2,000 IUs before conception. The larger dose should be taken during menstruation as this ensures that pregnancy has not occurred. Sugars should be eliminated from the diet because yeasts thrive on them. The local applicaton of yoghourt may also be helpful.

Chickenpox and shingles

Problems with chickenpox and shingles are rare because most women have established immunity to the virus, and because the virus does not tend to cross the placenta. However, in a very small number of babies born to women who do become infected, there seems to be a distinct pattern, including prematurity, skin lesions, neurologic anomalies, eye anomalies, skeletal abnormalities, gastro-intestinal and genito-urinary anomalies. (Alkalay 1987) Infections early in pregnancy may also lead to prematurity, stillbirth or miscarriage. (Brunell 1967) Other research has noted reduction and deformity of limbs, low birth weight and meningoencephalitis. (Savage 1973) High tone deafness occurred in one child, where the mother had been infected at 38 weeks gestation. (Aspock) It may be that some of these defects have been due to the deficiencies of zinc and manganese caused by the demands made on the immune system in fighting the disease, rather than the virus itself.

There has been concern about orchitis being associated with chickenpox, though only one case seems to have been reported in the literature (Wesselhoeft 1950) and at least one doctor has said that orchitis can probably occur with any infection. Even so, infertility does not necessarily follow. (Gray 1990)

Chlamydia

Chlamydia trachomatis is thought to be the most common sexually transmitted pathogen in the Western industrialised world. It is responsible for a great deal of sexually transmitted infection, as well as infertility, and ill health in infants.

(Schacter 1983) Since the symptoms are not always obvious the woman may not realise she is infected until her health is undermined. Chlamydial infection can be present for many years. One doctor reports a case of 22 years duration and of another who took a year to eradicate the infection before she was able to conceive. She had taken a fertility drug for a year without success prior to chlamydia treatment. (Sutton 1991) Testing as part of a preconception health check is therefore essential. More antibodies are found in infertile couples than in fertile ones. (Moore 1980)

In men, chlamydia causes between one third and a half of all non-gonococcal urethritis, although it often occurs with gonorrhoea. (Schacter 1983) It can cause inflammation of the prostate tubes, a painful and potentially sterilising infection, or even of the rectum, testes and vas deferens. In one study Chlamydia trachomatis, at 15.4 per cent, together with U.urealyticum at 15.8per cent, were the most prevalent microbiological findings in 209 male infertility patients. The researchers also found,

> "The inflammatory marker granulocyte-elastase was significantly increased in men with C. trachomatis: These men also showed significantly decreased citric acid levels indicating inflammatory damage of the prostate induced by C. trachomatis." (Wolff 1991)

This study also showed that the inflammatory response induced by the C. trachomatis is associated with reduced semen quality. In another study involving 326 infertile men, of the 136 who had clinical and microbiologically proved genital tract infection, the most frequent organisms found were gram-negative bacteria and chlamydia. (Minicic1990)

In women, it is a major cause of pelvic inflammatory disease, cervicitis, cervical cell dysplasia and urethral syndrome. (Mardh, 1981a) When it spreads from the cervix to the womb lining it may induce endometriosis. (Mardh 1981b) If it moves to the Fallopian tubes it can cause salpingitis which can result in blocked tubes and infertility. (Henry-Suchal 1980, Eilard 1976) If the tubes are partially blocked there is a risk of ectopic pregnancy.

One study has shown an incidence of 1.9 per cent among 7305 pregnant women. However, when the sample was restricted to women under 25 years of age who had at least one risk factor as identified in the study (young age or nulliparity or a new sex partner in the last year), 81.7 per cent were positive. (Alary 1993) A follow-up study of 30 women who had chlamydial infection at the time of an abortion showed that pelvic infection developed post-operatively in 63 per cent, with 7 out of 19 being admitted to hospital. The researchers concluded that,

> "Estimated costs of hospital admissions for complications of chlamydial infection were more than double the costs of providing a routine chlamydia screening program and prophylactic treatment."   (Blackwell 1993)

This does not take into account the emotional and financial costs of caring for a damaged baby born to an infected mother.

In children, at least 50 per cent of infants born to chlamydia positive women are likely to develop infections. (Munday 1983) One study quoted a 61 per cent rate of infections, with a 44 per cent rate of clinical disease in infants born to infected mothers. (Fromell 1979) Prematurity may result, and other main problems are conjunctivitis, found in 25-50 per cent of exposed infants, and pneumonia in 10-20 per cent. (Schacter 1979) Rhinitis, otitis media, proctitis and vulvitis have also been reported.

For example, in one study exposed infants had twice the rate of pneumonitis and recurrent otitis media in their first six months of life. Those who had pneumonitis had higher subsequent rates of gastroenteritis. The researchers concluded "these results suggest that appreciable outpatient infant mortality may be associated with maternal infection with chlamydia trachomatis and that it may either cause or promote the occurrence of early recurrent otitis media and gastroenteritis". (Schafer 1985)

Another study found Chlamydia trachomatis in the infant's pharynx and conjunctiva, the mother's cervix and the father's urethra. The researchers recommended searching for chlamydial infections in preterm infants with atypical respiratory disease even if delivered by Caesarean section. (Solletico 1987)

Coeliac Condition

This is a condition in which the sufferer cannot metabolise gluten, a protein found in wheat, barley, oats, and rye. It can cause severe physical and mental symptoms if it is not diagnosed, mainly because of the severe deficiencies arising from the malabsorption. Coeliac condition has been found to exacerbate infertility problems, especially in zinc deficient women. Treatment is by avoidance of gluten-containing grains.

Condyloma Accuninata (See Genital warts)

Cytomegalovirus (CMV)

Caused by one of the herpes viruses, this can have serious problems for men, women and infants. It is linked with low sperm count and inflammation of the testicle. (Alder 1984)

59

Prenatally it can cause miscarriage. Some 3,000 babies in the UK are estimated to be infected each year, 300 of them being left with a subsequent handicap. (Elek 1974) It is the most commonly known viral cause of mental retardation, though it may also be responsible for other conditions. (Hanshaw 1970) These include microcephaly, psychomotor retardation, developmental abnormalities, progressive hearing impairment, respiratory illness, jaundice, small for gestational age, failure to thrive and eye infections. (Blattner 1974, Dahle1970)

Genital Warts (condyloma accuminata)

Caused by the papilloma virus, the symptoms may only be warty nodules which may not be readily apparent. Some types of the virus have been linked with cervical cancer and may therefore affect reproduction. (Health Education Council 1985) By 1987, one in six women attending Islington , England, family planning clinics had a positive smear. One in three had either cell abnormalities and/or the cancer wart-virus. (Hollingworth 1987). (It is not clear how representative a group this is as compared with the general population.)

German Measles (Rubella)

This is not usually serious for the adult, but for the fetus it can have grave consequences. The dangers of abnormalities are about 50 per cent in the first few weeks of pregnancy, about 17 per cent in the third month, and almost nil thereafter. Some of the effects include congenital cataracts, deafness, heart disease, microcephaly, stunted growth, malformation of the teeth and low birth weight. There may also be miscarriages. (Rhodes 1961)

It would seem that there may be cumulative effects during life, if the fetus has been exposed to infection. In a study of 3,076 people who had been exposed, some of whom were 40 years old at the time of the investigation, the results confirmed a cumulative incidence of deafness to at least fifteen per cent by the age of twenty years. (Fine 1985)

Gonorrhoea

The bacteria Neisseria gonorrhoea-gonococcus is responsible for one of the most contagious diseases there is. Often the symptoms pass unnoticed, but if it is not treated gonorrhoea can have very serious consequences for men, women and infants. In men it can lead to sterility and low sperm counts. In the female it is a major cause of pelvic inflammatory disease, which may lead to sterility. It also seems to leave the woman more susceptible to chlamydial infections. (Cherry 1987)

If a woman has suffered from gonorrhoea, she is likely to be tested during pregnancy. At least one researcher has found that prolonged rupture of the membranes and later chorioamniocentesis in infected women predisposes the baby to acquire the infection. (Brooks 1985) There are also risks of prematurity in infected women. (Israel 1975)

Infections in the newborn are common if the mother is infected, as the bacteria are passed to the baby during its passage through the birth canal. Conjunctivitis is the most common problem, as the conjunctiva come in to contact with the infected cervix during birth – this can lead to a serious discharge with risks to sight, including blindness. (Brooks 1985)

Other parts of the body may also suffer, with infections of the umbilicus, the anogenital area, or nose and throat. There may be arthritis or meningitis.(Scarrel 1968)

Hepatitis B

At least two authorities have advocated universal screening for this condition, with vaccination as appropriate, because it is a serious condition leading to neonatal deaths. (Corbett 1987, Dulfer 1987) Another has argued that "the cost-benefit of screening is difficult to assess, but it is likely to be substantial". (Chrystie 1992) FORESIGHT recommends screening as part of the preconception care check. Hepatitis B can also lead to an increase in food and chemical sensitivities in the mother, which may affect a baby who is being breastfed. (Grant 1985)

Herpes

It is always advisable to ask if there is a history of herpes, since the patient may not be presenting symptoms at the time of consultation. A caesarian section may be advised where there is an active sore in the vagina or cervix. If the waters break a path is created for the virus to reach the fetus so a caesarian section must be done quickly. The virus may also be passed to the baby after birth by kissing if one has a cold sore or if there are sores on the breasts during breastfeeding. It is rare for the fetus to be infected in the womb and this would generally result in a miscarriage. (Sacks 1986)

Researchers have concluded that herpes "can result in spontaneous abortion, congenital and perinatal infections in the infant, or disseminated infection and death in the mother". The frequency of risk factors is unknown. In their study there was a 40 per cent incidence of serious perinatal disease or illness. Some infants whose mothers became infected in the first three months of pregnancy had perinatal morbidity such as prematurity, intrauterine growth retardation, and neonatal infections with herpes Type 2. (Brown 1987)

A main problem is that the baby's immature immune system may not be able to cope with the virus and this can lead to overwhelming infection, resulting in encephalitis with consequent brain damage, or eye infections, with eye damage. There may be jaundice, pneumonia with breathing difficulties, or even spells with no breathing at all. Microcephaly, microphthalmia and intracranial calcification have also been noted. There have been reports of physical impotence in men who suffered from herpes and proctitis, which then resulted in nerve inflammation. (Sacks 1986)

Influenza

There is some debate about whether prenatal exposure to influenza is associated with an increased risk of later schizophrenia. Some studies show no risk, while others show an association. In one study on 3,827 schizophrenic patients born in England and Wales between 1938-1965, the researchers found that females, but not males, exposed to influenza five months before birth have a significantly greater rate of adult schizophrenia. They cannot explain the gender difference. (Noritoshi 1994)

It is possible that deficiencies of zinc and manganese, due to immune system demands, could be the prime cause of the association. Boy babies have a five times greater demand for zinc than do girls. Boy babies would be more likely to be lost where the girls might survive.

Listeriosis

Caused by Listeria monocytogenes, an organism widely distributed in the environment, the most likely source of listeriosis infection for humans is food. In the UK in 1988, out of 291 reported cases, 115 were associated with pregnancy. Among these were 11 miscarriages, 9 stillbirths and 6 neonatal deaths. (Acheson 1989) Abortion, stillbirth or premature labour may occur soon after signs of maternal infection. Congenital listeriosis and acquired neonatal infection may present as pneumonia, septicemia or meningitis. Studies suggest that "up to a third of neonates may die and a third suffer long-term neurological damage". (Hay 1989) Another paper has reported about a fifty per cent mortality rate of Listeriosis infection occurs in the new-born period. (Gellin 1989)

Prevention: pregnant women should be advised to avoid eating soft, ripened cheeses (such as Brie, Camembert and blue-veined types) and commercially produced patés. Also ready prepared salads and unwashed vegetables. All cook-chill meals and ready-to-eat poultry should be heated until very hot. They should never be eaten cold. All manufacturers' directions should be followed completely.

Malabsorption

Malabsorption occurs as a result of other conditions such as allergies, infections, infestations, coeliac condition, candidiasis, nutritional deficiencies, toxic metal excesses, irritable bowel syndrome, Crohn's disease and colitis. Clearly if the patient is not absorbing nutrients properly, there are likely to be nutritional deficiencies which can affect pregnancy outcome. Mineral hair analysis and other tests can help to reveal a malabsorption problem.

Measles

"Measles during pregnancy can lead to fetal loss and prematurity, especially in the first two weeks after the onset of the rash" was the conclusion of a study of 58 cases. (Eberhart-Phillips 1993) With vaccinations, measles tends to be rather rare now, but this study has shown that it may still be a serious risk for the pregnant woman who is not immune.

Mumps

It is generally accepted that mumps can cause inflammation of the various parts of the sex organs, possibly leading to sterility or infertility. Research has suggested that mumps in the pregnant woman can affect the fetus later in life. An excess of diabetes was found among people exposed to the infection in the mother's womb in the first three months of pregnancy. By the age of thirty years, researchers had found a fifteen-fold increased risk of developing diabetes. (Fine 1985)

Mycoplasma Hominus and Ureaplasma Urea Lyticium

Among the smallest free-living pathogens, mycoplasma hominis and ureaplasma urealyticum are the most commonly cultured in the reproductive system. A direct relation between the frequency of venereal infection and serum antibody levels has been found. (Cassel 1986) One authority writes : "Mycoplasmas, which commonly reproduce when the subject's health is impaired, can cause attacks of vulvovaginitis, genital irritation and urinary frequency. Symptoms may persist for twenty years or even longer". (Sutton 1982)

In men, Ureaplasma urealyticum is a major cause of non-gonococcal urethritis, which can lead to infertility, non-specific urethritis (NSU), prostate and kidney disease. (Walton 1980, Grant 1988) Higher concentrations have been found in the genital tracts of sterile couples than in fertile couples. (Friberg 1973) In women pelvic inflammatory disease can result if the mycoplasmas, including Ureaplasma urealyticum, are allowed to proliferate. Scarring may lead to infertility. Miscarriage and premature birth are also associated with them. (Gibbs 1987) Of the common organisms Ureaplasma urealyticum is the most frequently implicated in repetitive abortions. (Simpson 1986)

Sutton has pointed out that genital mycoplasma infection is difficult to eradicate and prospective parents who have such a condition may have to be patient. (Sutton 1982) Women need local treatment of the cervix. Mycoplamsa are sensitive to antibiotics but develop resistance to it within days. Erythromycin and spiramycin were shown to have a better mycoplamascidal effect. (Mill 1979) Sutton has long pleaded for recognition of mycoplasma infection. "The unique quality of mycoplasmas is that they need steroids as an essential growth requirement, and hence they proliferate during pregnancy and when patients are given oral contraceptives or similar hormone drugs. It is because mycoplasma genital infection is not understood by both gynaecologists and STD clinics that the explosion in non-specific genital infection has occurred." (Sutton 1991)

He went on in the same presentation to explain that he uses a three stage antibiotic treatment for men: "five days co-trimoxazole, 48 hours break: three days metronidazole 600 mg a day, 48 hour break: ten days erythromycin 1-1+ gm per diem. For women I use a laser cautery procedure (an up-date on electro-cautery). All mycoplasmas are heat sensitive." (Sutton 1991)

Pelvic Inflammatory disease

This can be gonococcal, chlamydial, or non-gonococcal , non-chlamydial in type. It is sometimes misdiagnosed, so tests for all types should be conducted. Treatment for one type may be ineffective against another type. For example, antibiotics for gonorrhoea do not cure chlamydia. (Sutton 1982) One study found a high incidence of non-gonococcal infection among the male partners of women with PID. Over three-quarters of the males treated showed no symptoms. (Jacob 1987)

The consequences of untreated PID include sub-fertility, sterility, menstrual difficulties, chronic abdominal pain and ectopic pregnancy. (Grant 1985) The risks of tubal infection, including chlamydia, produced 12.8 per cent infertility rate, two infections produce a 35.5 per cent rate, while for three it is a 75 per cent rate. (Westrom 1975) Catterall reports: "If the statistics are correct there is a 50 per cent chance of relapse. . . , a one in three chance of being sterile, a 25 per cent chance of dyspareunia and a 10 per cent chance of an ectopic pregnancy." (Catterall 1981)

Syphilis

In both sexes, syphilis can lead to sterility and damage to many vital organs, including the heart and brain. It is transmitted from the mother to the fetus via the placenta, thus making it prenatal rather than congenital, though in the child it is usually referred to as "congenital syphilis". It only occurs when the mother's syphilis is not diagnosed and treated, making it comparatively rare in the UK and USA as most women's blood is screened at the antenatal stage. (Schofield 1972)

Without treatment one third of babies will be born healthy, though occasionally there may be a rash. However, failure to thrive and gain weight, often the first clinical signs of early congenital syphilis, become apparent two to eight weeks after birth. There may be weight loss, and often the baby has a wizened appearance, like an old man. Other symptoms include skin lesions, mucous membrane lesions, visceral lesions, enlarged liver and/or spleen, abdominal swelling, meningitis, and bone lesions. (Schofield 1972)

Toxoplasmosis

(We are grateful to Christine Asbury, Toxoplasmosis Trust, UK for allowing us to draw heavily from a talk she gave in December 1991.)

Toxoplasmosis is a condition caused by the parasite toxoplasma gondii. Toxoplasma are found in most animals, but only the cat is its reproductive host. It may be caught from cat faeces, raw or undercooked meat, contaminated and/or unwashed vegetables or fruit and unpasteurised milk and milk products.

30 per cent of 30 year olds and 50 per cent of 70 year olds in the UK will have been infected at some stage of their lives. 2 per thousand pregnant women will be infected during their pregnancy. In 40 per cent of them the infection will cross the placenta. 500 babies in UK are affected each year, 10 per cent being seriously damaged. Congenital toxoplasmosis can lead to hydrocephalus, blindness (through chorioretinitis), deafness, brain damage, mental handicap and epilepsy. The traditional triad is hydrocephalus, chorioretinitis and brain damage characterised by calcifications of the brain. A number of babies, usually those infected in the final trimester of pregnancy, may present as normal at birth, with the symptoms, particularly hydrocephalus and chorioretinitis, developing later, with a peak at aged 7 years. However it can be as late as 20 or 30 years of age.

Symptoms

In normal healthy adults, the infection is sub-clinical and most people will not realise they have had it. Symptoms may often be dismissed as those found in pregnancy: headaches, nausea, fatigue, sore-throat and flu. These should never be dismissed as a normal part of pregnancy.

Diagnosis/Screening

By blood test. This should be done during the preconception checks and subsequently throughout pregnancy. French doctors test at the preconception stage and at monthly intervals during pregnancy. The Toxoplasmosis Trust suggests at 12, 20 and 30 weeks during pregnancy would be an acceptable alternative.

Interpretation of test results is often confusing. A negative test will mean that the woman has never had toxoplasmosis and is vulnerable to infection during pregnancy. A positive test may mean that she has either had the test in the past and is now immune, or that she is currently infected. A second test should be done to see if IgG and IgM levels are rising, dropping or are stable.

If appropriate the woman may undergo a cordiocentesis between 20 and 22 weeks of pregnancy, and coupled with a scan, this should give information on whether or not the baby is infected and whether it has been damaged. However, final results of the test take about six weeks, though preliminary and fairly reliable results take two weeks.

Prevention

Pregnant women and those hoping to become pregnant should ideally never handle cat litter. Where they cannot avoid doing so, they should wear disposable gloves, wash their hands immediately after changing litter, change the tray daily and sterilise it with boiling water for 5 minutes each day: wear gloves while gardening: wash hands and implements thoroughly after handling raw meat, and do not eat raw or undercooked meat. Pink lamb is especially dangerous. Wash all fruit and vegetables thoroughly. Avoid unpasteurised milk and milk products, such as cheese.

Treatment

If a woman has a current infection the Toxoplasmosis Trust recommends that she immediately starts a course of antibiotic Spiramycin.

Any baby born to a mother thought to have been infected will be tested at birth. Clinical and sub-clinical infections should be treated, usually with pyrimethamine and sulphadiazine plus folinic acid. This is thought to prevent further tissue invasion and to reduce the risk of chorioretinitis. One expert and her colleagues in Turkey believe that early treatment with Pyrimethamine is successful in a significant number of cases. (Cengiz 1991)

Further information is available from the Toxoplasmosis Trust. (See Appendix one)

Trichomoniasis

Trichomonas vaginalis, a parasite of the uro-genitary system, is the cause of uro-genitory infections. With this condition, women may suffer from excessive, itchy vaginal discharge, although it is mostly asymptomatic. Men may suffer urethritis, prostatis and other urinary tract problems though they are generally asymptomatic carriers. (Murray 1990) The newborn child may have fever, irritability and may fail to thrive. (Corbett 1987)

Urinary Tract Infections

Bacteriuria infections include cystitis, pyelonephritis, and asymptomatic bacteriuria. Bacteriuria are detected in 2 – 10 per cent of pregnant women, a similar number in non-pregnant women. In non-pregnant women these infections frequently clear up spontaneously, but this is not so in pregnant women, where the clear-up rate is lower. If not cleared up with medical help, such infections can lead to spontaneus abortions. (Nicholas 1990)

A llergies – Food and Chemical

In 1906 Clement von Pirquet, a pioneer in the study of immunisation, defined allergy as 'observable altered reactions to environmental substances' (von Pirquet 1906). Since then the definition of allergy has become more refined. In his book in 1989 Jonathon Brostoff gave the following definitions:

> "Food Allergy is any adverse reaction to food in which the immune system is demonstrably involved.
> False Food Allergy denotes a special kind of nonimmunological reaction, seen with particular foods in which the food triggers the mast cells directly. The immune system is not at fault and the body does not overproduce IgE but the end result is the same with symptoms the same as allergy.
> Food Intolerance means any adverse reaction to food, other than false food allergy, in which the involvement of the immune system is unproven because skin-prick tests and other allergy tests are negative. This does not exclude the possiblity of immune reactions being involved in some way, but they are unlikely to be the major factor producing the symptoms.
> Food Sensitivity is employed as the umbrella term for all non-psychological adverse reactions to food.
> Food aversion means the dislike and avoidance of a particular food for purely psychological reasons."
>
> (Brostoff 1989)

Within the Food Intolerance definition some people may not react to a food for many hours, even days and so care must be taken when looking for allergies that intolerances are not overlooked because of the reaction delay. In a critical analysis of a study reported in the Lancet, (Lancet 1983) Jennifer Masefield has highlighted some of the study's weaknesses (Masefield 1988):

"Dried encapsulated foods used for double blind provocation tests may not give accurate results, because the actual state of the food may be the important factor. Some people can tolerate cooked cabbage but react to raw cabbage. The preparation of food can alter the allergen. Often certain food reactions are only caused by food combinations, so testing of foods in isolation will not produce a reaction. If an allergic person has not been exposed to an allergen for a long period he/she may have lost sensitivity to it. However, reactions may return after repeated exposures. In a multiple allergic patient who is repeatedly changing his/her diet to maintain better health, the sensitivity swing will make food allergy tests give different responses at different phases of the sensitivity level, for each excluded allergen or ingested allergen. This can give very confusing results, leading to an assumption of psychosomatic illness. If an allergen is excluded for only a few days, sensitivity is initially heightened and will show on testing."

FORESIGHT clinicians pay special attention to allergy for a number of reasons.

If a prospective parent is suffering from a food allergy, health is impaired, and there may be malabsorption which will generally lead to nutritional deficiencies.

Neglected allergies in either prospective parent seem to lead to allergies in their offspring, which can seriously impair development.

Clearing up allergies may mean that drugs do not need to be taken to alleviate the symptoms caused by allergens. Many such drugs are contraindicated during pregnancy.

Allergies may cause excessive mucus which can lead to blocked Fallopian tubes, a cause of infertility.

Investigating Allergy

There are a number of ways of investigating allergy, with varying degrees of effectiveness. We list below some of the main ones.

The clinical history is the most important and, ideally, should include reference to the wider family, especially the parents. Allergic symptoms, present in earlier life may alter and not be diagnosed as the cause of later problems found in, for example, the hyperactive, learning disabled child, the delinquent teenager and/or the aggressive husband who abuses his wife and children. (Bennett 1994)

Questionnaires can be useful in identifying symptoms. An example is given in Appendix three. (Masefield 1988) This extensive list of symptoms on the questionnaire unfortunately indicates why investigaton is so difficult.

A further example is the 'Medicmaster' questionnaire. (See Appendix one)

Cytotoxic blood tests, such as, the ALCAT procedure, performed by skilled technicians, are approximately 75 per cent reliable (ALCAT ~80 per cent) so can give useful guidance. (See Appendix one)

Skin prick tests and sublingual testing, which are sometimes used, are unreliable for food allergy.

Miller Provocation testing, a form of skin test, is more reliable and can be used to establish dosage for treatment.

Elimination and rotation diets are the most reliable methods. Many doctors specialising in ecological medicine (sometimes called clinical ecology or environmental medicine) put patients on a special diet to check for allergies. Depending on what the clinical history and questionnaires have revealed, it may mean cutting out all dairy produce and cereals, including refined carbohydrates. Basically this means eating meat and vegetables and the more unusual fruits such as pears. Often the patient will be asked to eat just lamb and game to start with, if it is suspected that beef, pork and/or poultry may be allergens.

Easier than this is just eliminating one food group and noting the effects. This is sometimes tried with the major allergens which are often the most commonly eaten foods and drinks in a particular country, such as wheat, yeast, chocolate, tea, coffee. eggs and milk in the UK.

If this does not improve the situation it may be necessary to try a rotation diet, designed to give each specific food only one day in five or seven days. An example of a rotation diet which has worked well with many FORESIGHT patients is given in Appendix four. It should be used in conjunction with a food diary, in which every food and drink taken is noted, with the time. There should be a separate column for comments, which will include any effects felt, either physical or emotional, and the times they were experienced. This is very important, since the reaction may not be immediate and so a list of likely causative agents should be gathered. It may be desirable to start the diary before the rotation diet with the comments column so that a primary list of suspect foods can be gained.

If allergens are found and removed from the diet it is important to ensure that the remaining components of the diet meet the patient's nutritional requirements. Allergies may change over time, or become a thing of the past if nutritional imbalances are sorted out.

The rotation diet (see Appendix four) is designed to give each specific food only one day in seven. The diet eliminates the most common allergens, cow's milk, grains and eggs. Also, all stimulants such as coffee, tea, chocolate and the sugars. No drink should be taken except the juice of the day and water. All foods must be boiled or steamed (in filtered or bottled water) or plain grilled or cooked in the oven in a covered dish. No fats, oils, gravies are to be used. During the trial period NO FOOD OTHER THAN THOSE LISTED MAY BE TAKEN AT ALL.

The diet will have ensured a fast of six days from any offending food so that the reaction to the allergen will probably be fairly immediate and may take the form of a running or stuffed-up nose, headache, stomach pain, feeling of bloatedness, extreme lethargy, irritability, etc. The day this occurs can be marked in the diet diary. It is then possible to test the foods eaten on this day one at a time.

Having thus worked out a basic diet of 'safe' foods, it will then be possible to test common allergens, such as cow's milk, eggs, the gluten grains – wheat, oats, barley, rye – and other fruits etc. After three weeks' abstinence the reaction may be strong, so at first only a small quantity of the substance should be given. If the reaction is very severe, a teaspoonful of bicarbonate of soda in water will help to alleviate the symptoms. After an adverse reaction, a return to known safe foods for a few days will be necessary before testing for another possible allergen. After a few weeks it should be possible to identify all food allergens.

The treatment of food allergies will depend on a number of factors, including how extensive the allergies are. It may be possible to get by with simple elimination. though this is no cure. There are various desensitising methods, ranging from drops to injections. A very practical and successful treatment which also covers chemical allergens is Enzyme Potentiated Desentisition, though as with all methods it does not work for everyone (Myhill 1991). Any doctor who is practising as a clinical ecologist, or using a nutritional approach in his/her work will be able to diagnose and treat the patient. Allergies to chemicals, such as food additives, pesticides and chemicals used in the workplace and home, may also be present. These are often difficult to diagnose and eliminate. (See Chemicals)

Most disease has some dietary aspect and will respond, at least in part, to nutritional intervention and the removal of toxins. This is especially true of the conditions discussed above, although it is not yet widely recognised.

A ssisted Pregnancy

However successful its programme has proved, FORESIGHT has always recognised that there will be some couples for whom more assistance is needed, maybe through in vitro fertilisation (IVF) or artificial insemination by husband (AIH) or by donor (AID). However, experience has shown that even in these situations, the preparation programme can enhance the likelihood of success.

IVF

Although IVF has assisted many couples to achieve parenthood, the procedure is still only approximately 20 percent successful. (Sweetenham 1994) The failures represent much misery and wasted expense for couples and anything that can be done to assist a successful implantation should be encouraged. Although a new technique has been developed which will enable only healthy eggs to be used, failure is still possible if IVF is forced on a body where the mineral levels are suboptimum. (See zinc and manganese in mineral section)

Ideally the couple should be advised to follow the FORESIGHT programme before referral for IVF, the referral only being made when the mineral levels are optimum, the infections are clear and toxins low. However, where one or both partners' hair charts are not optimised, but they are unwilling or unable to postpone an appointment for IVF they may be advised to continue the programme alongside any other treatment. Indeed, if they are receiving drug treatment, it is all the more important that they monitor their nutritional status, as the hormones given will raise levels of copper and lower levels of zinc. Hair mineral analysis should be done every three months and adjustments to their supplements made accordingly.

IVF is generally not regarded as suitable for women over 40 years of age, as it is said that the chances of a successful pregnancy after this age are very small. The FORESIGHT experience has shown that older women can have healthy babies of average or above average weight.

AIH – Artificial insemination by husband

Artificial insemination by husband is sometimes recommended when his sperm count is low. Although this procedure has been found helpful with about 30 percent of infertile couples, the FORESIGHT programme should be the first resort, as it seeks directly to improve the sperm count. Even if AIH has to be tried, a couple who have first followed the FORESIGHT program will be in better health, the sperm are therefore likely to be stronger and the female will be prepared for conception and a successful pregnancy.

AID – Artificial insemination by donor

Artificial insemination by donor is not without its risks, and although great care is taken to ensure the health of the sperm. There may still be problems, especially of infection. The FORESIGHT programme will ensure the optimum health for the woman prior to conception. It may also help the man, even by alleviating infertility in some cases. It should certainly be tried first in all cases where there is any sperm activity.

AID is always a difficult decision, with psychological problems for both partners often overlooked. (Prentice 1988) Even where the male partner becomes closely involved in the pregnancy and birth, as Winston says is his experience, it may still be a time of stress. (Winston 1986) With its emphasis on well-being, the FORESIGHT programme ensures the brain receives all the nutrients needed for a good mental state. (See section two on postpartum depression, which also applies to depression generally.) This may prove supportive.

Fertility drugs

As with all drugs these can compromise nutritional status (See Drugs). They should never be given without a full investigation of medical problems. It can be serious if hormonal treatment is given where there is a cervical or pelvic infection (See Adverse conditions). There has been some concern about the administration of fertility drugs without adequate monitoring which has resulted in some unexpected multiple births. (Public Eye 1995)

Chemical Hazards

> "Nearly every chemical to which the pregnant woman is exposed will ultimately reach the fetus." *(Spyker Undated)*

This section considers chemical hazards known or suspected of causing harm in reproduction. (A number of them are discussed under other sections – see Drugs, Food Adulteration, Pesticides and Toxic Metals.) Before looking at individual or groups of chemicals in more detail there are a number of general points that can be made:

1 The fetus does not have the mature immune system of an adult and is therefore less able to detoxify all the poisons that may be passed to it.

2 It is not easy to study the toxicological effects of substances, and many of the long-term effects are not known. Even where they are, it can be difficult to eradicate the offending substances – organochlorides and dioxin are good examples. Although DDT is banned in Britain and the USA it is still manufactured in these countries, then exported to the Third World only for them to export the food on which it is used back to Britain and the USA. Public analysts have found it in many foods.

3 Little is understood about the synergistic effects of chemicals. Toxicological tests rarely use protocols in which a group of chemicals is tested jointly, although this may be how they are used in practice.

4 It is unrealistic to eliminate all toxic substances from the home and workplace, but it is possible to limit their use, especially in the home. Professor Dennis Lincoln has linked chemicals such as those found in washing powders, cosmetics and detergents with falling sperm counts. (Nuttall 1994b) He also warned about oestrogen mimics in the environment. (See Food and Water adulteration) Friends of the Earth and Greenpeace are just two of the many organisations which can offer advice on alternatives.

The following list of chemicals is by no means exhaustive. Proven teratogens in the 1980s included:

Aminopterin	Procarbarcine
Antithyroid drugs	Phenytoin
Azathiopine	RetinoicAcid
Carbon monoxide	Thalidomide
Cocimadia	Trimethadione
Cyclophamide	Valproic Acid
Ethanol	Methyl mercury
Methotraxate	Daunrubicin

(Shephard, T H (1983)

(See also Appendix six)

Polychlorinated biphenols (PCBs)

Now banned in Britain, these were widely used in industry because of their specific properties, one of which was their resistance to biodegradation. This, unfortunately, has made them ubiquitous. They have been found in high quantities in semen samples and are now linked with low sperm counts, poor fetal growth, low birth weight, or poor survival rates. (Barlow 1982)

They are fat soluble so can be found in high concentrations in breast milk. (Mortensen 1986) The advice to mothers who are breastfeeding is to carry on, but not to try to lose weight while doing so, to avoid mobilising too much fat. The fact is that substitute milks are also contaminated, but they do not offer the other protective substances that human milk contains.

While they may be banned, PCBs are still found in old insulation systems and electrical appliances. PCBs penetrate human skin in less than half a second and even protective rubber gloves only help for four to five minutes (Saifer 1984) L-Ascorbic acid supplementation given to toxicated rats "afforded a definite protection against the enzyme activity alterations and histological changes caused by PCB toxicity." (Chakraborty 1978)

Vinyl Chloride

Widely used in more than half of all plastic products, these should not be confused with polyvinyl chloride, which has not yet been found hazardous except to people with chemical sensitivities.

Vinyl chlorides are linked with loss of libido in workers and a higher than usual incidence of neural tube defects has been reported in some towns with factories producing them, possibly reflecting damage to the sperm. (Norwood 1980)

There are also high numbers of fetal deaths, and wives of workers have a high rate of miscarriage. Decreased libido, impotence, decreased fetal growth, low birth weight and poor survival rates have been mentioned. They are known animal teratogens. (Elkington 1985)

Chloroprene

This has been linked with decreased libido, impotence, testicular damage, and infertility in the man and menstrual and other gynaecological disorders in the woman. (Barlow 1982)

Formaldehyde

This is associated with menstrual and other gynaecological problems, abortions, infertility, decreased fetal growth, low birth weight or poor survival. (Barlow 1982)

Solvents

Solvents include the aromatic hydrocarbons such as benzene and toluene. Many working women receive a double dose – at work and in the home. Some solvents are linked with decreased libido and impotence in the man, while in the woman some can cause menstrual and other gynaecological problems, with benzene being linked to maternal deaths related to pregnancy. (Barlow 1982) Benzene can damage the chromosomes and is possibly teratogenic. (Stellman 1979) The British Government published recommendations for limits to benzene in February 1994, mainly in response to fears about cancer. (Nuttall 1994c) It has been found that levels are higher inside cars than outside on a city street. (Ryan 1994)

Toluene has been linked with congenital abnormalities, particularly penile-urinary or genito-urinary defects. (HSA Undated a) Animal studies have shown an alarming range of problems, such as extra ribs, delayed development, retarded growth, hydrocephaly, and fetal death. (HSA undated b)

Solvents may also be a factor in decreased fetal growth, low birth weight and poor survival rates. (Barlow 1985) They were the presumed hazard in a Swedish study which reported that women in medical laboratories had more risk of spontaneous abortion and, perhaps, birth defects. They may also have been responsible for some spontaneous abortions among New York cleaners, although the stress of physical work could have been a factor too. (Chavkin 1984)

Perchloroethylene, an active ingredient in some solvents, is now under investigation in Britain, as it is suspected of miscarriages. It is already regulated in Europe and the USA. (Gardner 1994)

Methylene chloride, used in paint strippers, is linked with very low sperm count and shrunken testicles. (May 1992)

Dimethylformamide

Used in the production of paint, artificial fibres, drugs, leather dyes, pesticides and many other products, this chemical is linked with testicular cancer. (Lancet 1987)

Dioxins

Dioxins get into the food supply through pollution from chorine industries and incinerators. They are the most carcinogenic substances known (Saifer 1984).

Anaesthetic gases

A survey by the Americal Society of Anaesthesiologists found that nurses working in operating theatres had a 60 percent higher rate of deformed children compared with nurses in other departments, while female anaesthetists had twice as many deformed children as other female physicians. 25 percent more male anaesthetists had deformed children compared with other physicians. (Norwood 1980) Female dental surgeons have also been found to have high rates of miscarriage, probably as a result of exposure to anaesthetics, though dentists are generally at risk from mercury also. (See Toxic Metals) Fortunately it is possible to modify machines to reduce toxic emissions.

Carbon Disulphide

This is used in the manufacture of viscose rayon and as a fumigant. It is suspected of causing loss of libido, impotence and abnormal sperm. (May 1992)

Phthalates

Now under investigation by order of the British Ministry of Agriculture, Fisheries and Food, this group of chemicals is suspected of affecting male fertility. American research has found that they attack the Sertoli cells in the testes of rats. British research has found that they accumulate in fat tissues. The chemicals are used in printing inks and to make plastic more flexible. They are found in paints and cosmetics. They may leak into foods such as crisps and chocolates. (Nuttall 1994a)

Ethylene Bromide (EBD)

This is suspected of causing low sperm count and decreased fertility in the wives of workers who use it. It is used as an ingredient in leaded petrol (gasoline) and as a fumigant on tropical fruit for export. (May 1992)

Agrochemicals

Included among agrochemicals are pesticides (See Pesticides), fungicides, herbicides and artificial fertilisers.

The main problems with agrochemicals are that:

1 They do not treat the soil as a living organism but detroy its structure.
2 They harm the environment, indiscriminately killing organisms in the soil.

3 They adversely affect human health since the body is exposed to a multiplicity of new chemicals in amounts never before encountered by whole populations, and for which the body's detoxification systems were not designed.

4 The nitrates in artificial fertilisers are known "to alter and stabilise the chemical structure of haemoglobin, so that it is unable to bind and release oxygen". (Mansfield 1987)

Herbicides are often based on organophosphates (see Pesticides) and fungicides often contain mercury. (See Toxic Metals)

Contraception

Barrier Methods
Male Condom

Having fallen from popularity with the advent of the pill and IUD, the condom is now very much in favour because it is the only method of contraception which is recommended as offering some protection against sexually transmitted diseases, including AIDS, and possibly cancer of the cervix. Easily obtained, it is also the only method for which the man is responsible. It does not need medical advice or prescription and there are very few medical complications. Used properly it is a highly effective contraceptive, up to 98 per cent reliable, especially if combined with a spermicide to offer additional safety.

There are some problems associated with it, the most common of which are:

Not putting it on early enough, when genital contact has already been made;

Tearing it and not noticing, either during the process of putting it on, or inserting it in a dry vagina;

Using a lubricant which damages the rubber;

Letting it slip off during sex;

Letting it leak on the way out of the vagina;

Not being careful about avoiding contact between the penis and vagina just after it has been removed, when it is possible that there are still sperm on the penis.

Female condom

A female condom is now available but it is not cheap. It seems to have a higher failure rate than other barrier methods. (15 per 100 woman years.) Failure may occur when the penis misses the correct position and enters the vagina directly. It is visible outside the vagina and this may not be attractive to either partner. However, it may protect against infection and it is less likely to split than the male condom. The woman may also prefer to be responsible.

Diaphragm *(Also known as the cap)*

There are a number of caps, the most common being the diaphragm. Others include the cervical and vault caps which are held over the cervix by suction and they may be fitted where the diaphragm is unsuitable. The diaphragm is held by spring tension. All work by preventing the sperm from reaching the cervix, but since women's shapes vary so much and alter during intercourse, she should always use a spermicide. Correct fitting is essential and the doctor should ensure that the woman understands how to use it properly.

For the highly motivated couple caps can be very reliable – up to 97 per cent. Failure is normally associated with incorrect insertion or fitting, or defects through improper handling. It should also not be removed within six hours of intercourse having taken place. It may protect against cancer of the cervix. (Wright 1978) Since it can be inserted at any convenient time before intercourse, spontaneity is possible, although this means that some planning is necessary. There may be a loss of cervical and some vaginal sensation.

Sponge

This is a foam sponge impregnated with spermicide which can be inserted in the vagina up to 24 hours before intercourse. It must be left in for six hours afterwards to ensure that all the sperm are killed. It does not need special fitting and intercourse can be repeated within the 24 hour period, after which it is thrown away. It can, therefore, be expensive compared with other methods. It works by stopping the sperm from reaching the egg. Reliability, with careful use, is claimed to be up to 90 per cent. However, one study found a failure rate of up to 24.5 per cent. (McEwan 1986)

Spermicides

These work by the use of a base material which physically blocks the progression of the sperm, and a chemical which is designed to kill the sperm without irritating other body tissues. However, in some cases it may irritate one or both partners. Spermicides should not be used on their own. They are best regarded as a back-up to other barrier methods. Creams, jellies and foaming tablets are the preferred types.

Hormonal Methods
Oral contraceptive pill – *commonly known as the Pill*

It is likely that no other drugs have received so much attention as the oral contraceptive pills. It also probably true that much of the medical profession has never been so misled about a group of drugs, and consequently, has misled the general public. Because of this it is worth restating what the Pill is and how it works.

What the pill is

Oral contraceptive pills generally contain two synthetic hormones (steroids), oestrogen and progestogen, in various combinations according to trade name (the combined pill). The mini-pill contains just progestogen It can cause irregular bleeding and has a higher chance of pregnancy with its use. However, it really does not matter which type is prescribed, because hormones are injurious to a woman's health whatever the type and however administered.

How the pills work

Both oestrogen and progesterone levels in a woman remain high throughout pregnancy, thereby preventing the ovaries from preparing another egg to release. The combined pill works by confusing the body into thinking that it is pregnant by keeping the hormone levels high. Because oestrogen alone caused irregular bleeding, a progestogen was added to the pill. The commonly prescribed mainly progestogen pills make the cervical mucus thick and sticky and the lining of the womb atrophied and thin. Both of these actions increase the contraceptive effects, making it difficult for the sperm to enter the womb or for the womb to accept a fertilised egg. NORMAL MENSTRUATION IS PREVENTED. Thus when the pill is prescribed for painful or irregular periods, it works by stopping menstruation completely, because it stops normal ovulatory cycles. It then substitutes withdrawal bleeding when the pill is not taken for a few days each month. The cause of painful periods should be investigated before taking any action. Dr Ellen Grant maintains that painful cramps due to prostaglandin release may be part of a response to inflammation and using steroid hormones to suppress this natural response does nothing to treat any inflammation of the neck of the womb. (Grant 1988) FORESIGHT doctors find that in women of all ages, screening for/ treating genito-urinary infections and simple vitamin, mineral and essential oil supplements are a much safer way to relieve painful periods. They also carry no risk of interfering with the brain's control of ovulation.

Research

Of all the studies done on the pill the Royal College of General Practitioners' (UK) Oral Contraceptive Study is perhaps the most familiar. It was one of two large scale trials started in 1968. (Royal College of General Practitioners 1974) It is best regarded not as a clinical trial but "as a record of the natural history of two cohorts of women, one of which has used oral contraceptives while the other has not". (Kays 1984) Unfortunately it has erroneously been accorded the status of a proper trial, with the interim report quoted in the press as suggesting that the pill is a safe drug. Yet when the report is examined closely, there can be no conclusion other than one which points to the pill as a dangerous drug on the data available, without considering what damage could be inflicted in the long term. Sadly, since the 1974 report, there has not been a comprehensive follow-up.

Dr Ellen Grant has written a comprehensive critique of the study in *The Bitter Pill*, a book which gives a commendable overview of the problems associated with oral contraceptives. (Grant 1985) In it she explained that 47,174 women were enrolled on the study during 1968 and 1969. Even from the start the control and experimental groups were not randomised or equivalent. Obviously the experimental (pill-taking) group did not contain women in whom illness had already rendered the pill inadvisable, so this group was likely to be healthier than the controls. The drop-out rate from the pill-users group was large, even in the first three years. By 1979 it was enormous, with only a small percentage of the original pill-users group still taking the pill. The researchers had even switched 6,000 women in the control group to the pill-users (experimental) group to boost numbers. Why had so many dropped out?

Dr Grant believes that the "big exodus was hardly surprising as the 1974 report showed a large number of medical conditions were increased in pill users. . . an increase in over sixty conditions."

She presents evidence to show an increase in many of these, for example, in suicide, cancer and vascular conditions. (Grant 1985) Her detailed review to the British Medical Journal complaining that "the high drop-out and side-effects rates did not justify further use of the pill" was cut to a short letter. (Grant 1988)

She also pointed out that the study did not measure total morbidity, as was claimed. It measured only conditions that the doctors recognised – and there are a number of important conditions that many doctors do not always acknowledge, such as some allergies and widespread nutritional deficiencies.

Dr Grant is not alone in her concern. As far back as 1969 Williams wrote:

> "In fact, the pill has been shown to be capable of affecting any or all systems and organs in the body, with a great variety of consequences."   (Williams 1969)

In the same year, Barbara Seamans wrote:

> "Very few pill-users have the slightest notion of the potency of the drugs they are ingesting, or how the little pills may affect their own health or their still unborn children."   (Seamans 1969)

In 1974 Dankenbring wrote an overview of the dangers of the pill, including quotes from eminent doctors to a Congressional subcommittee. (Dankenbring, 1974)

The risks associated with the pill

Dr Paavo Airola, a world authority on nutrition and biological medicine has listed risks to health associated with the pill under two headings: the less serious, which are still bothersome, and those which cause serious complications. (Airola 1979) One can argue with his divisions – depression and increased susceptibility to vaginal and bladder infections when one is dealing with preconception care are hardly "less serious", but taking both lists together one can gauge the detrimental effects to female health. His lists include:

"Less serious, although bothersome"

Increased susceptibility to vaginal and bladder infections.

Lowered resistance to all infections.

Cramps.

Dry, blotchy skin. Mouth ulcers.

Dry, falling hair, and baldness.

Premature wrinkling.

Acne.

Sleep disturbances.

Inability to concentrate.

Migraine headaches.

Depression, moodiness, irritability.

Darkening of the skin of the upper lip and lower eyelids.

Sore breasts.

Nausea.

Weight gain and body distortion due to disproportional

distribution of fat.

Chronic fatigue.

Increase in dental cavities.

Swollen and bleeding gums.

Greatly increased or decreased sex drives.

Visual disturbances.

Amenorrhoea.

Blood sugar level disturbances which complicate diabetes or

hypoglycaemia.

"More serious complications"

Eczema.

Gallbladder problems.

Hyperlipemia.

Intolerance to carbohydrates leading to "steroid diabetes",
which can lead to clinical diabetes.

Strokes.

Seven to ten times greater risk of death due to blood clots.

Jaundice.

Epilepsy.

High blood pressure.

Kidney failure.

Oedema.

Permanent infertility.

Varicose veins.

Thrombophlebitis and pulmonary embolism.

Heart attacks.

Cancer of the breast, uterus, liver and pituitary gland.

To this list one can add:

Vitamin and mineral imbalances.

Ectopic pregnancy.

Miscarriage.

Food allergies.

Genito-urinary disease, including cervicitis.

Congenital malformations in offspring.

Osteoporosis.

Ovarian and lung cancer. (Grant 1988, Grant 1985)

Fungal infections.(Grant 1994)

Although there have been claims that the pill protects against ovarian cancers there are still concerns about breast cancer and blood clots (Hawkes 1994b, Hawkes 1994c, Drife 1994, Greenhalgh 1995a)

The instructions for the use of the pill list many of the above as contra-indications, warnings or side effects. The small print may not be easy to read, but if one perseveres, one can see that the "information" is presented very cleverly to minimise the adverse picture painted. For example, in one set of instructions for use it is claimed that, "Painful periods are in most cases abolished," implying that the user still has periods. Throughout the instructions the words "period" and "bleeding" seem to be used interchangeably, implying that a woman's periods continue when on the pill. Nowhere does it make clear that menstruation ceases absolutely. The side effects are referred to as "occasional," which is not what Grant and others have found. The user is advised to stop taking the pill immediately pregnancy is suspected "since it has been suggested that combined oral contraceptives, in common with many other substances, might be capable of affecting the normal development of the child in the early stages of pregnancy." Does this advice not rest uneasily with the warning earlier in the instructions that "Not even the combined oral contraceptive can offer 100 per cent protection against pregnancy." Since malformations can arise very early in pregnancy, stopping after the pregnancy has been recognised will, in many cases, be too late. In view of what is known about the effect of hormones on the fetus, it is nonsense. The teratogenic effects are underestimated because of the number of miscarriages which occur. (Cilag 1994) (It is interesting to note that earlier instructions for this same pill mentioned the words "fetal malformation" and said, "It can be definitely concluded, however, that if a risk of abnormality (fetal malformation) exists at all, it must be very small." (ORTHO-NOVIN)

The most important aspects affecting preconception are considered in more detail below and elsewhere in this book. However, it should be remembered that anything which affects the health of the mother can indirectly, if not directly, affect the health of the fetus.

The pill and vitamin and mineral imbalances

The pill upsets the balance between copper and zinc levels in the body, raising copper and lowering zinc. This can be very serious as zinc is one of the most widespread mineral deficiencies in the Western world. Often therefore, when a woman comes off the pill to become pregnant she will start a conception in a zinc deficient state, which will get worse as the pregnancy progresses. This can lead to problems during gestation for mother and fetus, as well as problems for mother and infant after birth. Difficulties may include post-natal depression and lactation problems in the mother and feeding difficulties, learning difficulties and developmental difficulties, especially with regard to sexual development. Excess copper has been associated with pre-eclampsia and post-partum depression, among other conditions. The pill interferes with other minerals, especially magnesium, iron, iodine and probably chromium and manganese. (Grant 1985) (See Minerals)

Nor is vitamin metabolism left unscathed. As Grant says: "Steroids change protein building and breakdown in the liver and change the levels of protein in the blood that carries the vitamins to the body tissues. The pill can alter the actions of the enzymes which need vitamins to function properly." (Grant 1985) The pill raises Vitamin A levels and leads to deficiencies of B1, B2, B3, B6, folic acid and C. It may lower B12.

Ectopic pregnancy

Ectopic pregnancy has now reached epidemic proportions in the USA and is increasing in the UK. (Polan 1986) Even where the pregnancy can be successfully aborted, the woman will often have severe Fallopian tube damage or even lose the tube. Some women may have low magnesium levels which may impede tubal muscular action. Some may have infections. There may also be high copper levels. (Grant 1988)

Miscarriage
Pill users have a higher risk of miscarriage even after they have stopped taking the pill, unless specific mineral and vitamin levels are restored to normal.

Food allergies
These are dealt with in detail elsewhere. Grant believes that the pill is a major contributory factor in the increase in food allergy which has now become serious. (Grant 1985) This is not surprising when one remembers that the pill compromises the immune system leaving it less able to cope with sensitivities. Its effects on liver function mean that enzymes which should help in detoxification are inhibited, thereby exacerbating the effects of toxins from foods and chemicals to which an individual may be allergic. Nutritional imbalances, especially zinc deficiency, are major factors contributing to allergy.

Genito-urinary infections
These are also dealt with in detail elsewhere. Suffice to say here that the pill has led to an increase not only through greater sexual freedom, but also because of its physical effects on the body. It weakens the immune system so the body is not so resistant to infection. It has led to increases in cancers, especially of the cervix in younger women. In part, this is because it was given to many of them when their bodies were still growing, their cervix linings were still immature and susceptible to changes, particularly those leading to cancers. (Grant 1985)

Congenital Abnormalities
Since Dr Isabel Gal first discovered that hormone pregnancy tests (which are no longer used) were associated with higher incidences of congenital malformations of the central nervous system, studies have continued into the teratogenic effects of the pill and other hormones. (Gal 1967) Some researchers have claimed that recent studies have not confirmed an association, (Harlap 1985, Royal College of General Practitioners 1976), although there are others spanning three continents, which have found statistically significant numbers of abnormalities. In the USA, researchers found limb-reduction anomalies in one study, with major abnormalities, including congenital heart anomalies and neurological and neural tube disorders in another. (Nora 1975, Nora 1978) These findings were confirmed in a major study in Europe, as well as in a number of small ones. (Hellstrom 1976, Janerich 1974) In Australia, researchers concluded that "the relative risk for a limb defect, was 23.9." (McCreadie

1983) However, when the results of this study were subjected to a more stringent statistical analysis, the risk was 30.2. (Kricker 1986) Other researchers argue that, "Hormonal treatment during pregnancy may be a predisposing factor in congenital heart defects." (Levy 1973) Even researchers of studies which failed to find links warn that there is a need for further studies. (Mullvihill 1974, Oakley 1973)

Fertility

The pill interferes with the hormone system to prevent pregnancy. However, after a woman has ceased taking it, the body's systems may not return to normal. Having had the message to switch off making certain hormones for so long, the body takes time to adjust to producing them again. Sadly for some women, the adjustment may take a long time, or may never happen. Nutritional imbalances, especially zinc deficiency are also often a factor. The FORESIGHT experience is that the full FORESIGHT programme will often restore ovulation.

Intra-uterine devices – *the IUD or coil*

It is still not clear how the IUD works, though it is known that its continued presence in the womb prevents conception. It may prevent the egg from attaching to the lining of the womb by mechanical means, or it may be by some toxic action. Its failure rate is higher than the pill. It is also quite harmful, the side effects including :

Cramping and pain, especially during menstruation.

Ectopic pregnancy.

Spontaneous abortion.

Uterine bleeding.

Blood poisoning.

Bowel obstruction.

Cervical infections, infection of the uterus and of the Fallopian tubes.

Pelvic infections.

Dysplasia.

Cancer of the uterus.

Anaemia.

Perforation of the uterus.

It can become imbedded in the uterus, which often means hospitalisation and can even mean death.

Mineral imbalances, especially elevated copper and low zinc.(Airola 1979)

In an attempt to overcome some of these problems, sometimes chemicals, such as progesterone or progestogen, are added. As the section on the pill has shown, this is not a safe practice. Many of the side effects are caused or exacerbated by poor fitting. Users cannot check it is in the correct position.

Drugs

In discussing drugs, this section takes a broad view, including social drugs, such as tea, coffee, cola, cigarettes, alcohol, over-the-counter and prescribed drugs, as well as those banned by law. ALL drugs have side effects and in prescribing, the doctor consciously and conscientiously weighs these against the benefits. Yet too often the patient overlooks the need to consider balance when taking social drugs.

Factors common to all drugs

It does not matter what the drug is: it will always have an effects on the body's chemistry which is not natural. Reviewing the literature on how drugs and chemicals adversely affect the offspring of mammals Dr Justin Joffe, Professor of Psychology, University of Vermont, concluded that, regardless of the species of animal, the chemical given, its dose, and its timing, there were three main effects which seemed common to many studies: smaller litters, lower birth weights in those animals actually born, and higher mortality rates in the newborn. (Joffe 1979) During pregnancy it is now recognised that the placenta does not act as a barrier across which toxins do not pass. Substances, as the Thalidomide and DES tragedies showed, can reach the fetus with devastating consequences, although there may be some ways in which protection is offered by the mother. Drugs can also reach the baby through the mother's milk. (Committee on Drugs 1983, Broadie 1986, Elkington 1985)

Although there are compulsory tests which drugs have to pass before going into use, there is doubt over the effectiveness of the tests. At least one statistician has claimed that the basic test method may give the wrong result in 50 per cent of tests. (Salsburg 1985) Moreover, the tests do not always consider synergistic effects of taking two or more substances simultaneously. The dangers to the user of mixing alcohol and sleeping tablets are well known, but the dangers to the fetus of most combinations of drugs are not usually discussed. Adverse reactions are sometimes magnified when two or more substances are taken together, though this will depend on a number of factors, including the drugs themselves. (Beaulac-Baillargeon 1987) Babies born to mothers who smoke marihuana and drink alcohol have been found to have a greater risk of fetal alcohol syndrome. They are at greater risk of low birth weight. (Mann 1985) Caffeine-cigarette interactions have also been associated with low birth weight. (Beaulac-Baillargeon 1987) Some of the effects are indicated in the drug information, which will list contra-indications. This is why it is important for the doctor to be aware of ALL the drugs a patient is taking.

It is in the area of nutrition that drugs are probably most detrimental. Drugs affect nutrients in a number of ways. They can lead to impaired absorption as, for example, when laxatives form a physical barrier to fats by dissolving them before the body can ingest them. Others, such as mineral oil, may absorb essential nutrients which are then excreted. They may compete with nutrients at the gut wall and the nutrients may lose the fight. They can cause increased excretion of nutrients that the body needs. Alcohol is a classic example, causing excretion of a number of nutrients, including some B vitamins, zinc and magnesium. Yet others may lead to redistribution of nutrients in the body at the cellular level or increased requirements of certain nutrients. They may even decrease nutrient requirement, as in the case of the pill and iron. To add to the complexity of all this, they may do a number of these together. (Buist 1984)

Prescribed and self-prescribed drugs

Ideally both parents should not be taking drugs before conception, and the female should not be taking drugs during pregnancy or breastfeeding, but there will be situations in which the doctor considers it essential. It is advisable to inform the patient of any side-effects and drug-nutrient interactions and to offer recommendations to minimise the adverse effects. It has been found that when people are given a diet appropriate to their personal nutritional needs, and have their deficiency and allergy problems cleared, they can often reduce their medication to a lower dose or even to nil. Another therapy, such as relaxation, may also be beneficial.

It seems likely that the teratogenicity of drugs is frequently related to the drug/nutrient interaction. It has been suggested that the Thalidomide tragedy may have been due to riboflavin (Vitamin B2) deficiency. (Robertson 1962) In experimental animals, this deficiency produces malformations like those suffered by the Thalidomide victims. Thalidomide resembles riboflavin in chemical structure and could therefore have blocked the uptake of the vitamin.

Some diabetics have responded well to dietary intervention using vitamins and minerals and have been able to reduce their insulin dose. Many food additives and pesticides have been implicated in the causation of epilepsy, as has a deficiency of manganese. (Underwood, 1977, Pfeiffer 1983, Passwater 1983, Aston 1980, Duffy 1979, Duffy 1980)

Alcohol

Although there is now little dispute about the existence of fetal alcohol syndrome, there is still considerable disagreement about how much alcohol it is safe to drink. (Plant 1987) An expert on early embryology, Professor Matthew Kaufman has explained that it is impossible to advise on a safe limit, adding that "the only thing we can say is safe is none at all until child-bearing is over, though presumably that would be totally unacceptable socially." (Kaufman 1988) The Surgeon General of the United States has stated: "Pregnant women, and those planning a pregnancy, should abstain from the use of alcohol." (US Surgeon General 1981) Neither of these authorities address the issue of male drinking, although FORESIGHT believes that there is sufficient research data to take the following position:

> NO alcohol in the preconception preparation phase for both partners, and during pregnancy for the woman.

Alcohol travels through the blood stream to affect the sperm, egg and fetus. One animal study gave male mice alcohol for 26 days, then sobered them up for two days before breeding. The litters produced had only half the normal number of pups, and only 12 per cent of them survived more than a month. (Anderson 1988) Kaufman has found that serious chromosome faults appear in up to 20 per cent of mice embryos after only moderate doses of dilute alcohol. He believes that since alcohol has a specific effect on the chromosomes, ingestion is one of the major factors in thousands of miscarriages, as well as in many of the babies born with mental and physical handicaps. (Kaufman 1988)

Male drinking habits are often overlooked, yet this acceptable social drug is known to affect the sperm. In heavy drinkers the sperm often lack normal tails, which will affect sperm motility. (Van Thiel 1975) Two researchers were able to predict, statistically, a decrease of about 137 grams in infant birth weight if the father had an average of two drinks or more daily, or at least five on one occasion in the month leading up to conception. (Little 1987) Russian research has also suggested sperm abnormalities in alcoholic fathers can cause fetal abnormalities.(Shurygin 1978) Tuormaa's excellent review gives further evidence of the effects of alcohol on male reproduction. "Alcohol is a direct testicular toxin." (Van Thiel 1975) It causes atrophy of semeniferous tubules, loss of sperm cells, and an increase in abnormal sperms.(Bennett 1950) Alcohol is also known to be a strong Leydig cell toxin and it can have an adverse effect on the synthesis and secretion of testosterone. (Lipsett 1980, Ylikahri 1974, Mendelson 1978) Alcohol can cause significant deterioration in sperm concentration, sperm output and motility. (Kucheria 1985, Brzek 1987) Semen samples of men consuming excessive amounts of alcohol have shown distinct morphological abnormalities. (Dixit 1983, Wichman 1992) It has also been established that approximately 80 per cent of chronic alcoholic men are sterile and that alcohol is one on the most common causes of male impotence. (Van Thiel 1974, Master 1970) (Tuormaa 1994 – booklet available from FORESIGHT) See table 8 for effects of alcohol.

The Maternity Alliance (UK) published an earlier review, written by the Wynns, of research on the damage caused, such as higher spontaneous abortion rates, more stillbirths, reduced fertility and more abnormalities. (Wynn Undated) Basically children of drinking mothers show physical abnormalities that fall into four categories:

1 Central nervous dysfunction, with mental retardation of varying degree. In some children IQ may be low, although in others it may be average, but they have learning problems, such as poor attention span.

2 Growth deficiencies, being of low birth weight, and short at length at birth. Normal post-natal growth does not happen.

3 Facial abnormalities, with distinct features, including low nose bridge, narrow upper lip, small chin and a flat face.

4 Other malformations, especially heart and dental defects.

Other researchers refer to defects of the mouth, genito-urinary system, hernias and birthmarks, as well as a weak ability to suck. (Streissguth 1979) Where a number of these are found in the same child, he/she may be identified as a victim of fetal alcohol syndrome. It has also been suggested that there may be hyperactivity, distractibility and short attention span. (Cooper 1987)

The Fetal Alcohol Study Group drew up a set of minimal criteria for diagnosis of this syndrome, covering specific aspects of growth, the central nervous system and characteristic head and facial features. (Rosett 1983) It is difficult to assess the incidence of the syndrome, since definitions vary. One authority quotes at least one in 600 to 700 children, though in some communities with high alcoholism rates, it may be as high as one in a hundred (May 1991).

Patients who do not display enough features to be regarded as having the full FAS are often called Fetal Alcohol Effects (FAE) or "possible FAE" if they have a clear history of alcohol exposure. They are still at risk of brain damage even without the physical features of FAS.

The potential effects of alcohol on brain development are regarded as the most difficult. When giving the 1990 Betty Ford Lecture, Dr Ann Streissguth, a world authority on FAS, said,

"Now, after 17 years of clinical experience with such patients, it

**Table 8 : Male Hair Zn Concentration and Alcohol Consumption
– 367 subjects (Ward 1993)**

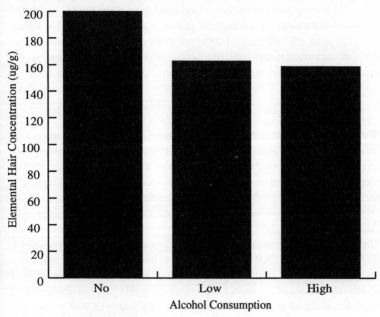

**Table 9 : Hair Fe Concentration and Alcohol Consumption
– 367 subjects (Ward 1993)**

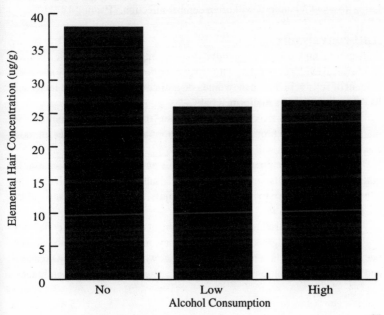

has become all too clear that the accompanying psychopathology is the primary long-term outcome of Fetus Alcohol Syndrome. Management of the behavioural problems is the biggest challenge to their care. Their medical problems are not trivial. . . No matter how difficult these medical problems might be to deal with, they are small compared to the behavioural management problems presented by many of these children, particularly as they enter puberty."   (Streissguth 1991)

She elaborates on their behavioural problems, which include anti-social behaviour, difficulty learning from normal experience, troubles holding jobs and training, and problems with the law. Any drinking, even social, before pregnancy recognition or during pregnancy is a risk to the fetus. See table 9 for effects of alcohol consumption on iron levels in the hair.

Antibiotics

There seems to be general agreement that antibiotics have been over-prescribed, with the serious result that they have ceased to be effective in some situations, though there is continuing disagreement about their possible adverse effects on the micro-flora of the bowel. No antibiotic should be prescribed without careful consideration of the alternatives, as they interfere with normal gut metabolism. They are of no use in viral infections and can seriously weaken the immune system, especially if use is prolonged or frequently repeated. Large doses of Vitamin C will often combat infection. (Pauling 1971)

Anti-convulsants

Anti-convulsant drugs, especially dilantin and phenobarbitone, induce biochemical evidence of folate deficiency if the diet contains a barely adequate amount of folic acid. Pregnant women on anti-convulsants have an increased likelihood of having a malformed baby.

The FORESIGHT experience has been that when magnesium and manganese levels are brought to within the normal references ranges, in most cases the convulsions will cease.

It may then be possible to discontinue anticonvulsant medication. In other instances convulsions may respond to an anti-allergenic diet. Unless the convulsions are known to be due to a head injury, it would seem wise to adopt the FORESIGHT approach.

These drugs also increase the requirement for Vitamin D. A deficiency of this vitamin is dangerous during pregnancy and in the child who is being breastfed there could be a risk of rickets. Other work suggests that manganese and magnesium and the amino acid taurine can help stabilise cell membranes.

Anti-depressants

Anti-depressants which are monoaminase blockers are known to decrease sperm count and motility. (Blair 1962. Davis 1966) Tricyclic anti-depressants do not have the same effects. Depression will often respond to the cessation of the use of social poisons and the restoration of trace mineral status, especially zinc, magnesium, manganese and B complex. (Pfeiffer 1978)

Aspirin

Claims about an association between aspirin-taking, low birth weight and a high perinatal mortality rate have come from Australia. (Collins 1975, Turner 1976) The findings were not confirmed in two US studies, although the subjects were taking smaller doses. (Stone 1976, Shapiro 1976) A study looking at aspirin use and subsequent child IQ and ability to concentrate found that use in the first half of pregnancy was significantly related to a lower IQ and inability to concentrate in those children who had been exposed to aspirin in the womb. (Streissguth 1987) It is therefore very worrying that the Medical Research Council should have considered a trial using aspirin to lessen the risk of pre-eclampsia. (Fletcher 1988, Greenhalgh 1995b) The FORESIGHT experience is that pre-eclampsia has not yet occurred on the FORESIGHT programme.

Beta-blockers

Research has shown that the male is not immune to side effects of drugs which may interfere with his fertility. (Soyka 1980, Editorial, British Medical Journal 1964) Phelezine, a beta-blocker, decreases sperm count and motility. (Davis 1966, Blair 1962)

Caffeine

> "The sufferer is tremulous and loses his self-command: he is subject to fits of agitation and depression; he loses colour and has a haggard appearance. The appetite falls off, and symptoms of gastric catarrh may be manifested. The heart also suffers; it palpates, or it intermits. As with other such agents, a renewed dose of the poison gives temporary relief, but at the cost of future misery." (Allbut 1906)

This is how the authors of a medical textbook in 1906 described the caffeine addict. However, it is rare for a doctor to ask about caffeine intake, though this alkaloid drug is widely taken in tea, coffee, soft drinks, foods and medicines. It has an initial stimulating effect in small doses and can temporarily relieve fatigue. It also raises blood pressure and stimulates the kidneys. Five or more cups a day is reckoned to be an addictive dose, though not everyone drinking this amount will become addicted. (Wetherall 1981) Most people will ingest more than this in their food and drink unless they check carefully. The doctor may wish to advise patients to keep a food and drink diary.

Most research on its effects on both male and female reproductive systems is not encouraging. In certain amounts it can affect sperm motility, with large amounts causing complete immobilisation.(Wetherall 1981, Mohsen 1983) Consumption during pregnancy has been associated with abortion, chromosomal abnormality and congenital multi-abnormality and late spontaneous abortion. (Furuhashi 1985, Wichit 1985)

Since it appears in many foods and beverages, patients should be advised that the only certain way of avoiding it is to buy fresh foods and do their own baking, watching the ingredients. Decaffeinated is not recommended, as it contains other stimulants, and possibly harmful residues such as pesticides. (Saifer 1984) (See pesticides)

Cocaine and Crack

Animal studies have reported that cocaine is teratogenic in mice even at non-toxic levels.(Mahalik 1980) Rats showed higher resorption rates and a significantly lower fetal weight. (Fantel 1982) These findings have been replicated in human studies. A study of three groups of women, 50 cocaine only abusers, 110 multi-drug abusers, and 340 non-drug users concluded that "Cocaine abuse in humans significantly reduces the weight of the fetus, increases the stillbirth rate related to abrupto placentae, and is associated with a higher malformation rate". The babies suffered mild withdrawal symptoms. (Bingol 1987) Use of the drug in early pregnancy is a risk factor for congenital heart defects. (Morris 1992) It has been linked with congenital urogenital anomalies. (Chavez 1989)

The cocaine-derivative, crack, is much more addictive and is more rapidly absorbed into the vascular system. Besides the same risks as cocaine users, babies born to minority heterosexual populations of US crack users have been shown to be at greater risk of congenital syphilis, emphasing further the need for genito-urinary screening for all. (Crane 1992) Withdrawal symptoms in the new-born are severe.

Heroin

Heroin, in common with other opiate drugs, such as morphine, opium and codeine, is known to lead to decreased fertility and atrophy of the male accessory sex organs. They also decrease testosterone. (Smith 1985) In women addicts there are many complications during pregnancy. They have a three times greater risk of stillbirth than non-addicts, a four times greater risk of prematurity and a six times greater chance of a baby suffering growth deficiency. A significantly higher number of infants with congenital abnormalities can be seen. There are also higher rates of jaundice and respiratory distress syndrome. Low birth weight and small size for gestational age are found. There is an increased perinatal mortality, with rates up to 37 per cent in some studies. Other fetal complications noted include infections and episodes of stress. There may be long-term effects on growth and behaviour, with regard to perceptual and organising abilities. (Ostrea 1979, Naeye 1970, Wilson 1979) The babies are born addicted to the drug and have to undergo the stress of withdrawal.

Hormones

Sex hormones used therapeutically in pregnancy may cause malformation of the fetal sex organs, as well as aberrant behaviour. Taken during delivery, they may affect the neonate's weight gain and response to nursing. (Brazelton 1970) (See Contraception)

Hormones have proved especially hazardous for the unborn child. The first synthetic hormone, Di-ethyl stilbestrol (DES), was found to cause cancer in children after their mothers had been given it during pregnancy. Yet more hormones were developed,though they are banned in many European countries because their effects are not fully understood. Britain, Canada, the USA, France and Ireland are the only countries to permit all five hormones sold on the international market. However, a ban does not mean they are not used. Research has shown that growth promoting hormones, banned in Europe, are still used in the beef industry all over Europe. Natural hormones are banned in Europe but permitted in the USA. (Consumers Assocation 1995)

Controversy is still raging over the use of BST – bovine somatotrophin, a hormone given to stimulate milk production in cows. BST is currently banned in Britain, and the ban is likely to continue until 2002. A MAFF spokesman confirmed that it causes mastitis in cows and its effects on human health have yet to be confirmed (MAFF 1994a). Thus it is not yet known if BST can pass through breast milk and therefore into the baby. Any connections with breast cancer, undescended testicles, ovarian cysts in female fetuses or low sperm count, to mention but a few health problems, have yet to be researched. Given our knowledge of the injurious effects of the contraceptive pill, it seems incredible that the Government may be prepared to expose people or the unborn child to exogenous hormones without being certain of their effects on health. The only guarantee of avoiding BST if it is permitted, and other growth promoting hormones, is to use only organic products.

Hypertension Medication

Anti-hypertensives may depress sperm count. (Winston 1986)

Marijuana – *pot, cannabis*

Research suggests that marijuana is four times more dangerous than cigarette smoking, because the smoker inhales more deeply and holds the breath for longer. (Anon 1987) This results in three times more tar in the lungs and five times more carbon monoxide. Tetrahydrocannabinol (THC), the psychoactive substance in marijuana, has the steroid structure found in the sex hormones and certain hormones of the adrenal gland. THC tends to accumulate in the ovaries and testes. In women it upsets the menstrual cycle, though it is possible to become tolerant to it, in which case the cycle is restored.(Mann 1985) In men heavy use of 5 to 18 joints a week for six months has been noted to cause a marked lowering of blood testosterone, lower sperm count, greater than usual impotency and diminished libido. (Elam 1980) Sperm motility is also affected and there is an increase in the number of abnormal sperm. (Mann 1985)

The drug has been shown to affect the synthesis of DNA and to slow the growth rate of cells. (Mann, 1985) In animals it has been linked with an increase in fetal deaths and malformations. (Sassenath 1979) In humans it is likely that babies will be smaller because of the increased carbon monoxide levels, which will make less oxygen available to the fetus. It induces chromosomal damage. (Strenchever 1974) There seem to be dose-related behavioural effects, which occur in all babies born to mothers who are heavy abusers. Prolonged or arrested labour may occur. (Mann 1985)

Medication for Morning Sickness

Often women who have followed the FORESIGHT programme do not suffer much discomfort from morning sickness. Anti-nausea medications should certainly be avoided, as the Thalidomide tragedy showed. For those who feel they need a remedy Dr Harold Buttram suggests that drinking 6 to 8 glasses of unpolluted water daily will help in many cases. (Buttram 1994) (See Section two Infertility) Ginger is also a harmless antidote.

Smoking
(See tables 12 and 13 re number of prospective parents)

The dangers to health of smoking are still the subject of much debate but there can be no dispute that smoking during pregnancy is a major cause of abnormal- ity, avoidable illness, handicap and deformity in children. (US Public Health Care Service 1980) Female smoking is linked with infertility. (Campbell 1979) Babies born to smoking mothers are, on average, 7 ounces lighter than those born to non-smoking mothers, though this weight reduction may not be significant. (Simpson 1957) The reduction in growth is mostly due to hypoxia, but nicotine itself causes decreases in uterine blood flow and placental amino acid uptake.(Crosby 1977) Naeye reported abnormally large areas of dead tissue in the placentas of mothers who smoked or had done so. (Naeye1979)

Such damage to the placenta interferes with the nutrition of the fetus. Cadmium, an inorganic poison present in smoke, becomes concentrated in the placenta. Cyanide, also present as a result of the hypertensive effect of thiocyanate, interferes with fetal nutrition, impeding growth and leading to low birth weight. (Grant 1986, Abel 1983) Heavy smokers and drinkers have a six times greater risk of stillbirth. (Goujard 1978) Heavy smokers also have a higher risk of spontaneous abortions and fetal malformations, including cleft palate, hare lip, and central nervous system abnormalities. (Himmelberger 1978) There is a higher incidence of premature births and short-for-date full-term infants in smokers. (Fedrick 1976, Miller 1976) There seems to be a greater risk of tubal pregnancy for current smokers, compared with women who have never smoked. (Chow 1988) It is possible that minor brain damage may be caused. Studies have shown poorer learning abilities and behavioral problems in children born to smokers compared with those born to non-smokers. (Abel 1983, McGee 1994)

This is not surprising given that there are over 4,000 known compounds in tobacco smoke. Nicotine, the addictive substance, is the most widely known. Besides the effects already mentioned, it has been shown to lower hormone levels in animals, which may affect fertility and milk production. (Hawkes 1994d) It also interferes with nutrient absorption in the fetus. Nor are passive smokers free from risk to their fetus, especially if they are in smoky atmospheres for long periods. Carbon monoxide, released by burning cigarettes and cigars, builds up in the atmosphere. High levels lead to a reduction in the oxygen-carrying capacity of the blood, depriving the fetus of an optimum level of oxygen.

The effects of male smoking can be serious. German workers have reported that the fetus can be affected by the amount the father smokes. Where the father smoked heavily, the child was more than two-and-a-half times more likely to have malformations. Facial malformations were related to the smoking level in the man. Smoking lowers testosterone levels, and affects sperm count, spermatogenesis, sperm morphology and sperm motility. (Mau 1974, Kulikauskas 1985, Rantala 1986, Briggs 1973, Evans 1981)

Children of smokers have higher rates of illness, particularly respiratory infections, and increased risk of cot deaths. Intellectual, physical and emotional development is slower than in children of non-smokers. (Grant 1986)

Although there is not yet agreement among experts, some are suggesting the existence of a fetal tobacco syndrome. They claim there are certain features common to children born of heavy smokers. (Nieburg 1985) Smoking is known to cause changes in the appearance of adults, and in a study of the appearance of new-born infants, medical and nursing students were able to distinguish correctly, in significant numbers, between those born to smoking and non-smoking mothers based on intuitive selection. (Stirling 1987)

Table 10 : Male Alcohol and Smoking History – 367 subjects (Ward 1993)

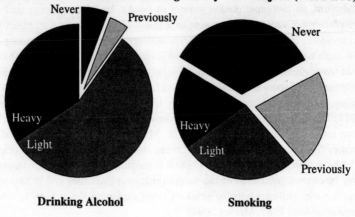

Drinking Alcohol   Smoking

Table 11 : Female Alcohol and Smoking History – 367 subjects (Ward 1993)

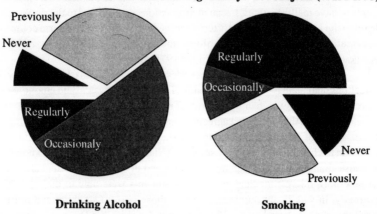

Drinking Alcohol   Smoking

Table 12 : Hair Cadmium Concentration and Smoking Activity – 367 males (Ward 1993)

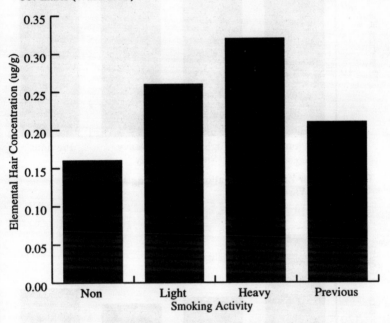

Table 13 : Hair Iron Concentration and Smoking Activity
– 367 males (Ward 1993)

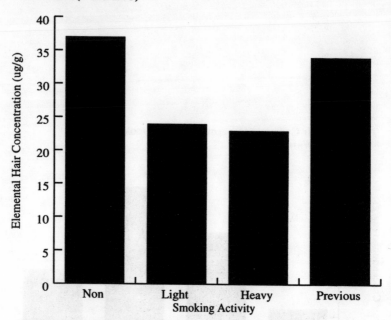

Table 14 : Hair Zinc Concentration and Smoking Activity
– 367 males (Ward 1993)

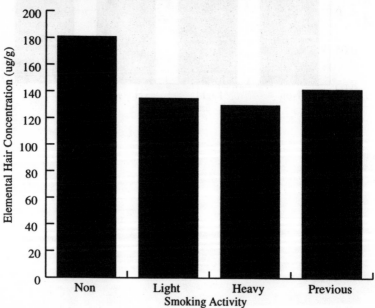

For those readers who want to make a more detailed investigation of the effects of tobacco on reproduction, Tuormaa has written on excellent review. (Tuormaa 1994 – booklet available from FORESIGHT.) See tables 15,16 and 17 for effects of smoking on cadmium,iron and zinc levels in hair.

Tranquillisers and Sleeping pills

Benzodiazepines should be avoided at any time during pregnancy. They have been linked with visible malformations, functional deficits, and behavioural problems in exposed children. They can disturb the central nervous system in the very early stages of pregnancy. (Weber 1985) Other researchers have suggested that mothers who take them during the first three months of pregnancy are 3.3 times more likely to have a baby with an oral cleft. (Rodriguez 1986) In many cases, tranquillisers are taken to counteract the effects of over-stimulation by other social drugs , such as excessive coffee or the effects of deficiencies such as zinc, magnesium, manganese and B complex vitamins, which can be easily corrected once recognised.

Withdrawal from substance abuse

As all doctors know, withdrawal from substance abuse is never easy and addicts can sometimes be quite difficult to work with. However, there are some general points that may help in treating such patients. The main thing to remember is that no addict will have a healthy body – they will always have biochemical or physiological imbalances as a result of their abuse. Indeed, these imbalances may initially have provoked the addiction.

It is advisable that a full biochemical screening is undertaken following which the doctor can provide the patient with a programme to re-balance the body. This will involve a detoxification programme to remove toxins. Vitamin C and other nutrients can be used for this. (See toxic metals and hair mineral analysis.) Acupuncture is also useful in detoxification. Detoxifying means not abusing other addictive substances, including sugar, coffee, tea, coke, and other caffeine-containing drinks.

A useful programme for overcoming substance abuse which the doctor can encourage his/her patient to follow with the doctor's support is given in Dr Keller Phelps' book, *The Hidden Addiction*. (Keller Phelps, 1986) Besides re-balancing and detoxifying, the doctor can encourage the patient to take exercise, eat a nutritious diet, learn about their addictive substance (it is amazing how ignorant most addicts are of the health effects of their substance), find new activities, take counselling and keep a positive attitude.

The doctor should warn pregnant addicts against sudden withdrawal, as this can precipitate an abortion or premature labour. (Royal College of Psychiatrists 1985) The doctor should also warn against sudden withdrawal from certain drugs, including prescribed ones.

Food and Water Adulteration

The adulteration of food occurs at every stage of its life cycle, from the start of its growth to the period when it is processed in or out of the home before being eaten. Agrochemicals, which are second only to genetic manipulation as the initial stage of adulteration are discussed elsewhere in greater detail, as is the benefit of organic foods. (See Pesticides) Here we shall look at the value of whole grains, additives, the commercial processing of food and water.

The value of whole grains

The 1983 report of the National Advisory Committee on Nutritional Education (NACNE) recommended increasing the amount of whole grains in the diet, not only because this would lead to an increase in dietary fibre, but also as it was "more likely to ensure increased intakes of minerals, trace elements and other micronutrients; elemental malabsorption is also less likely." (Health Education Council 1993) Why are whole grains a better food?

Taking wheat as an example, the question can be answered by considering what happens to the grains in the processing. The whole grain has three main parts: the outer layer, or bran; the germ; and the inner section, or endosperm. When the grain is milled to make white flour, the bran layer and 75 per cent of the germ are lost, leaving the flour consisting mostly of the endosperm. (Davies 1981)

But the parts lost contain most of the micronutrients needed by man. As one expert wrote:

> ". . . the milling of refined white flour removes 40 per cent of the Chromium, 86 per cent of the Manganese, 76 per cent of the Iron, 89 per cent of the Cobalt, 68 per cent of the Copper, 78 per cent of the Zinc and 48 per cent of the Molybdenum, 60 per cent of the Calcium, 71 per cent of the Phosphorus, 85 per cent of the Magnesium, 77 per cent of the Potassium, 78 per cent of the Sodium. . . "
> (Schroeder 1973)

Valuable vitamins are lost also, among them being B1, B2, B3, B6, Pantothenic acid, Folic acid and E. B1 is particularly necessary for metabolism of carbohydrates such as wheat. Where it is absent in the food, the body will draw on its precious reserves from the central nervous system in order to metabolise the food for the energy it requires. During processing a few of these vitamins are replaced in small amounts, with each country having its own preferences. In addition, millers are required to add certain minerals. In Britain, for example, iron is added, though in a poorer form than that removed, and calcium in the form of chalk which is not a normal source. When the flour is made into bread, various additives are also permitted, including bleaching agents, improvers, extenders and preservatives. Again there is variation between countries. (Brady 1986)

The dangers to health posed by 'enriched' flour were demonstrated by Dr Roger Williams in an experiment with rats. He fed one group 'enriched' flour and another group the same flour but with many more added nutrients to make it similar to wholemeal. After 90 days, of the rats fed the 'enriched' flour "about two thirds were dead of malnutrition and the others were severely stunted". (Williams 1973)

Not only is white flour deficient of essential minerals, it may also contain high levels of cadmium. In refining the flour, zinc, which tends to be found in the bran layers, is lost, leaving the cadmium found mostly in the centre of the grain. Cadmium is able to displace zinc in strategic enzymes and inactivate them. (Ballentine 1978)

Some experts worry about a substance called phytate in flour, arguing that the phytate which is retained in wholemeal but lost in the refining, binds up zinc and carries it out of the body. The problem is compounded because the enzyme which destroys the phytate needs zinc. However, fermenting the bread with yeast increases the availability of zinc, because it seems to produce enzymes which destroy some of the phytate. (Ballentine 1978) Unfortunately most bread today is not produced by fermenting yeast. Moreover the practice of adding extra bran to the dough can further exacerbate zinc deficiency by adding extra phytate. Home baking your own is the best way! Phytate in meusli can also be reduced by soaking the grains in water overnight. (Jervis 1984)

'Pure, White and Deadly'

This is the description of the substance which was considered the most addictive there is by the late Professor John Yudkin, a world authority on sugar. (Yudkin 1986) Raw sugar, made from sugar cane juice by just evaporating the water and allowing it to solidify and granulate, is dark brown and sticky, because of the molasses it contains. These molasses are a rich source of trace elements which are necessary for the metabolism of sugar. When sugar cane or beet is processed to give white sugar, all that remains is sucrose. Most of the trace minerals are lost, including "93 per cent of the Chromium, 89 per cent of the Manganese, 98 per cent of the Cobalt, 98 per cent of the Zinc and 98 per cent of the Magnesium." (Schroeder 1973)

Food Additives – including the 'E' numbers.

There are now about 4000 additives in use in the UK though only about 350 of them appear on labels. (Millstone 1988) Not all are permitted by other countries, who accept scientific evidence suggesting they pose a health hazard to some people. What are they and why are they necessary?

Additives which have been reviewed by the EC Scientific Committee on Food and deemed safe for wide use are given an 'E' which then appears in the list of ingredients. Unfortunately toxicological tests that the chemicals undergo do not reveal all the possible adverse effects, nor are combinations of chemicals as they appear in foods subjected to testing. Comparatively few additives are required to be listed. As two leading experts wrote:

> "In reality, less than 10 per cent of all additives are ever listed on labels. . . At least 3,500 flavourings are used, and this entire class of chemicals is exempted from these labelling regulations. At most a product may list "flavourings" on the label, but it is never stated whether one or 50 are being used, much less give their names."
> (Millstone 1988)

Not all additives are artificial, though this is not always understood. A few are derived from natural products, including some colours and vitamins.

The most common additives are salt and sugar. In some foods so much sugar is added that it becomes the main ingredient, even though it may be disguised as such by the multiple of names it goes under: glucose, maltose, fructose, lactose, sucrose, dextrose and golden syrup, to mention but a few. (Cannon 1987) Patients anxious to avoid additives of questionable safety may be advised to buy the guide book *Find Out* available from FORESIGHT.

Processing

The amount of processing depends on the final market product. Thus, some fruit and vegetables will be sold in the form in which they were harvested. However, some of it, especially apples and pears, will be subject to some processing, such as waxing, to help it travel and store in a 'good' condition. Storekeepers argue that the customer likes to see a shiny apple, equating this with quality. 'Perfect' foods, such as those sold by large retailers, can only be produced by the use of agrochemicals and careful marketing techniques.

The major purpose of most processing is to add monetary value. A good rule to apply is that the more monetary value added, the more nutritional value lost.

Many processed foods, cakes, biscuits, breads and 'sweets' are made from cheap ingredients and/or artificial ingredients, and therefore do not contain the level of nutrients in the home-made equivalent. If an item is cheaper than the home made version, it is usually because it is made from inferior ingredients, and is loaded with additives to disguise this.

When it comes to meat, the food technologists have produced a new range of products which is sold to the customer legitimately as 'meat'. Such products include Mechanically Recovered Meat (MRM), obtained by machines which strip flesh off bones. Meat, according to the 1984 Meat Products and Spreadable Fish Products Regulations, means 'the flesh including fat, and the skin, rind, gristle and sinew in any amounts normally associated with the flesh used, of any animal or bird normally used for human consumption and includes any part of the carcass specified in Part 1 of Schedule 2 which is obtained from such an animal or bird, but does not include any other part of the carcass'. Reformed meat may be shaped into 'steaks', or the poorest quality meats may be used in pies and other products. (Cannon 1986)

Antibiotics

In 1988 Sir Richard Body MP, former Chairman of the Agriculture Select Committee, warned that excessive use of antibiotics in animal feed was producing strains of salmonella to which there may be no check. (Body 1988)

As long ago as 1953 the drug companies secured a change in the law to permit penicillin and chlortetracycline to be used in feedstuffs as a growth stimulant, although it remained illegal for humans to have either except on prescription. Two years later oxytetracyclin was allowed and the quantity of antibiotics consumed by farm animals increased steadily from then on.

By the 1960s it was noticed that some strains of Salmonella pyphimurium were resistant to antibiotics when 14 children in Yorkshire died of salmonella poisoning. This lead to an inquiry by a committee chaired by Sir Michael Swann which divided antibiotics into two groups; one for therapeutic use only and one which could be used as growth stimulators. Unfortunately the law which was passed, based upon Swann's report, is doomed to failure because of the similarity between antibiotics. If salmonella, or any other microbiotic organism, were to acquire an immunity to one antibiotic no-one can say that it will not be able to adapt that immunity to other antibiotics with a very similar chemical composition.

As the demands for enhanced growth and profitability from each farmed animal grow and the use of antibiotics as growth enhancers increases to match them, then the likelihood of more resistant strains of micro-organisms developing will also increase.

Preserving Foods

Man has preserved foods for centuries – and some of the methods are still in use, such as drying and salting. Once sugar was discovered to be a preservative it too became popular. Advancing technology brought new methods, including freezing and canning. Food ceased to be preserved as a necessity in case of seasonal shortages. Tinned foods, and later on frozen ones, became cheap enough for everybody, often cheaper than fresh food, and with the advantage of a longer period of availability. With tinned peas, for example, you could eat them all year. What was overlooked was their inferior nutritional value. Freezing meat destroys 70 per cent of the pantothenic acid : in vegetables over half the B vitamins are lost. Canning is worse! Tinned peas and beans have lost over 75 per cent of pantothenic acid and vitamin B6. For green vegetables the figure is over 50 per cent. Tinned tomatoes have had 80 per cent of their zinc removed, while carrots have lost 70 per cent of their cobalt. Storing the cans for a long time results in further losses of about 25 per cent. (Colgan 1982)

Irradiation

Food irradiation is a process by which food is exposed to high level of gamma radiation to kill microscopic bacteria, thus increasing the shelf life of items such as grains, meat, herbs, spices, fruit and vegetables. Unless there is an error in the equipment or by the operator, the food does not become radioactive. However, electrons in the chemicals making up the food are knocked out of orbit and massive molecular rearrangement occurs. Free radicals are formed. Vitamins A, D, C, E, K, B1, B2, B3, B6 and folic acid are depleted or destroyed. Some amino acids are broken down, fats go rancid and carbohydrates create very toxic chemicals. New chemicals are formed called Unique Radiolytic Products (URPS), most being unknown and none has been adequately tested.

Irradiation does not make food safer – quite the reverse. It does not kill botulism, though it does kill botulism's natural enemies, thereby leaving the way open for botulism to thrive. Food which is 'off' will not have a warning smell. Other disease-producing organisms will be mutated, while aflotoxin, a highly carcinogenic compound produced by moulds, is produced in higher quantities. It does not reduce the use of chemicals in foods, and no one knows what it does to their residues. In fact, it increases the use of chemicals to counteract the changes in texture, smell and flavour produced as a result of the process.

The British Medical Association is firmly opposed, arguing that it could put children's health at risk. Where animals have been fed irradiated foods adverse effects have included tumours, cataracts, chromosome breakage, kidney damage, fewer offspring and higher mortality (Webb 1985). The only certain way to avoid eating irrradiated foods is to consume organic products.

Storage

Finally, storage of crops can also bring dangerous side effects to the consumer. Ideally grains should be sun dried after harvesting. Florence Nightingale always insisted that "wheat, barley, oats, maize and millet purchased for the army in India must be freshly harvested, be clean and have a moisture content of under 10 per cent." (Ramsay Tainsh 1984) If grains are not dried off properly, moulds may develop, which may produce harmful substances called mycotoxins. These can cross the placenta and may induce abnormalities in the fetus, depending on how advanced the pregnancy is.

H air Mineral Analyses, Supplementation and Cleansing
by Belinda Barnes

Mineral testing, followed by supplementation and cleansing programmes where indicated by the results, is arguably the most important aspect of preconceptual preparation. (Ward 1993)

As is shown throughout this book, a weight of scientific evidence in published books and papers has demonstrated the link between trace mineral deficiencies and/or high levels of toxic metals, and all types of reproductive anomaly. (Jennings 1970, Price 1945, Pottenger 1983, Underwood 1977, Oberleas 1972, Hurley 1969, Hurley 1976, Pfeiffer 1978, Vallee 1965, Saner 1985, Passwater 1978, Williams 1973, McCarrison 1984, Laurence 1980) If the whole huge volume of scientific data is applied in a programme of preparation, then babies are conceived and carried in optimum conditions, in a nutrient-rich, pollutant-reduced environment. Under these circumstances they thrive and flourish, as the FORESIGHT experience has demonstrated.

Infertility and in utero death, perinatal death, prematurity, low birth weight, malformation of the fetus and postnatal illness in the young have been eliminated or reproduced at will in many species of experimental animal and in livestock breeding. Isobel Jennings, MRCVS, when a veterinary pathologist at the University of Cambridge, described the lack of fertility and the malformations seen in the young of experimental animals denied the necessary levels of vitamins in utero. Many of the vitamins and essential fatty acids work synergistically with the minerals. For this reason, FORESIGHT gives a full vitamin and essential fatty acid supplement alongside the mineral programme.

The follow-up of human tragedy has been studied. In response to lead contamination in particular, differences in brain function, postnatal growth rate, and in the survival of the baby, have been noted. (Wibberley 1977, Bryce-Smith 1977, Ward 1993, Bellinger 1978, Bellinger 1987, Schroeder 1971)

This section focuses on hair mineral analysis, looking at a range of typical hair charts with their analyses, and the use of supplementation to re-balance the body, supplementing deficiencies and removing toxins. Charts and supplement lists may be found at the end of the section.

Typical problems encountered include:

a) A chart with a general scatter of low or borderline levels of nutrients (such as magnesium or zinc) with or without some raised levels of toxins (such as lead or aluminium).

b) A chart with the low minerals even more marked, with perhaps four or five below the normal range. The reasons for this may include poor diet (junk food), over-enthusiastic slimming regimes, ingestion of toxic metals, allergy, malabsorption due to undiagnosed coeliac condition or intestinal parasites. (See Allergy, Toxic metals, Intestinal Infections and Adverse conditions)

Charts 1 – 12 show different aspects of multiple deficiencies, and typical programmes designed to overcome them.

c) A low level of zinc with a high level of copper. This pattern in women usually follows the use of oral contraceptives, the copper IUD, or super-ovulatory drugs such as Clomid, Pergonal, and others. (Pfeiffer 1978, Grant 1994) Over-high copper will cause premature birth or miscarriage. (Vallee 1965) This may explain the very high rate of early births with Clomid pregnancies, including those following IVF. To raise the zinc and lower the copper levels under these circumstances may take rather heavier supplementation with zinc than would be the case with a lower level of copper (hair level of under 20 ppm). Manganese and selenium will also help the copper to retreat a little. The ideal copper level for the start of a pregnancy is 15–20 ppm.

Charts 2, 5 and 10 and their programmes demonstrate this.

d) Low zinc on its own, or among a scatter of other low levels, may be the result of a refined carbohydrate diet, the pill, illness, surgery, emotional trauma or heavy metal toxicity. (Schroeder 1971, Pfeiffer 1975, Grant 1994, Bryce-Smith 1984) Urinary tract infection can squander zinc through diuresis. In addition to supplementation, it is as well to evaluate, and where possible eliminate the causes of zinc deficiency. (See Adverse conditions)

Charts 1,2,3,4,5,6 and 10 show very low levels of zinc.

e) Low manganese may be due to pesticide contamination. The choline-containing enzymes are needed for the transfer of manganese across the gut/

blood barrier and these are immobilised by the organophosphate pesticides. (Pfeiffer 1983, Underwood 1977, Passwater 1983, Jennings 1970) (See pesticides)

Charts 1,2,3,7,8 and 10 refer.

f) Low magnesium has also been linked to pesticide contamination and to fluoride in the water. Fluoride complexes with magnesium and renders it unavailable to the body. Artificial fertilisers, based on nitrogen, phosphorus and potassium, are also said to make magnesium less available to plants (grains, vegetables and fruit). Magnesium deficiency is quite commonly seen. (Ward 1993)

Charts 1,6,8 and 9 refer.

g) Low selenium is also quite commonly seen. The cause for this may be stresses on lung function. Selenium is known to be helpful in retaining integrity of the lungs. It is therefore possible that passive smoking, traffic effluent, industrial contamination or spraydrift of agrochemicals may play a part. Low selenium has been linked by American research to Downs syndrome so it is vital to ensure a good hair level before the start of the pregnancy. Selenium is also used by the body to cleanse aluminium and other toxins which are often present in drinking water.

Charts 1,2,3,4,5,8,10,11 and 12 refer.

h) Low nickel is demonstrated by the work of Forrest Nielson to be a causative factor in heart defects in the unborn.(Nielson 1984a and 1984b) As with all trace minerals, an excess can also be harmful. For this reason nickel supplements are unavailable. It is to be hoped that, following further research, this decision will be reversed in the future. Meanwhile we have to rely on some little amount being obtained from kelp supplements.

Charts 1,2,3,5 and 7 refer.

i) Low chromium and cobalt often appear together where there is heavy consumption of sugar or alcohol, or in the case of low cobalt, vegetarianism. (Schroeder 1973, Pfeiffer 1978) A stable chromium is essential to prevent diabetes. Either deficiency may also appear alone.

Charts 1,3,10 and 11 refer to both minerals.
Charts 4,8 and 9 refer to low Chromium only.

j) High levels of a toxic metal. (See Toxic metals) A water filter is mandatory. FORESIGHT recommends both a cleansing programme per se, and the use of the balancing minerals, ie those said to help the elimination of the toxin. EDTA or penacillamine are not recommended as both these preparations can also strip beneficial minerals from the body.

Aluminium and lead are quite hard to eliminate as they may be stored in the bone. At the start of the programme stores may be released into the blood, thus at this stage the hair levels may rise rather than fall in the repeat hair chart. Couples should be warned that this may happen otherwise there can be disappointment. If the toxic metals are not eliminated before conception, there is a risk that a pregnancy will release the stores into the body due to hormonal influences. Thus a large dose of stored pollutant could be delivered to the baby at a moment of maximum brain development. It should be suggested to couples that they are particulary rigorous with contraception while mobilising and eliminating the toxins.

For cleansing we use Vitamin C-with-Garlic, and the liver cleanser HEP 194 in cases showing very severe contamination.
In cases showing high levels of toxins a series of essential minerals can also be used. (Bryce-Smith 1981, Pfeiffer 1978, Lodge Rees 1984)
For lead: calcium, iron, manganese, and zinc are helpful.
For cadmium: chromium is helpful. (Schroeder 1971)
For aluminium: magnesium and selenium are helpful.

Charts 2,3,4,5,6,9,10 and 11 refer.

If toxic metals are high, or copper over-high due to artifical hormone use, then mineral supplements may need to be increased. An increase in the level of the beneficial mineral will often help to reduce the level of the toxin or the excess copper. Zinc, maganese and selenium will balance up copper.

The single minerals can be used with the usual base of 2 FORESIGHT vitamins, and 2-4 FORESIGHT minerals. In borderline cases the number of FORESIGHT minerals should be taken into consideration.

Some minerals compete for binding sites in the gut (eg zinc, selenium and manganese). (Underwood 1977, Pfeiffer 1975, Passwater 1983) We therefore normally give them at separate times. However, the programmes are often more successful if all the minerals are present at some time during the day. (This raises the question as to whether the binding sites are programmed to receive each mineral only after a small stimulus from a balancing mineral. It would seem logical as it would provide some form of crude homeostasis.)

However, it is not a difficulty as small amounts of the balancing minerals will be present in foods and in the FORESIGHT Minerals. Balancing mineral supplements more specifically may speed things up, however, if large changes are desired very quickly.

Magnesium and potassium need to be kept in balance. Significant supplementation of one will lower levels of the other. Supplementation of both may be helpful unless there is already a discrepancy that needs to be corrected.

Too much iron can be toxic. Iron in the blood can vary through the day. Supplementation should be light. FORESIGHT advises 7mg or 14 mg a day, and for a short time only (eg one to three months), with Vitamin C to help absorption.

Programmes should be given for 4 or 5 months, and then the hair should be retested. Couples often need to be reminded to retest. They should be advised not to start a pregnancy if the levels are not satisfactory.

It is necessary to warn couples that levels may not be perfect by the retest. Everybody's metabolism is different and sometimes optimum levels may be elusive. However, the more closely they stick with the full programme and dietary guidelines, the greater the chances of success, sooner rather than later.

It is a common problem that one partner, usually the woman, is keener to comply. It can be very frustrating for one partner if their retest shows improvement, with levels that would be suitable for pregnancy, but there are still hazardous deficiencies in the other partner. This may need to be pointed out in advance.

Some couples feel they will be able to do it all "by diet". Unfortunately sixteen years of experience has demonstrated that this is unlikely to be successful within the timescale of 4 to 5 months, if at all, but a retest should be recommended in any case, so their progress can be monitored.

FORESIGHT gives all couples:
Their hair data;
Their supplement programme;
The letter of instruction;
The address of Vitamin Service;
The Wholefood Diet Leaflet;
The Natural Family Planning Leaflet;
The Leaflet on the Avoidance of Toxic Metals;
The form for retesting hair.
If they have not received them previously we also give them the WHY leaflet, the fliers for the books and the video, and the booklet *Preparing for Pregnancy*.

In the follow-up consultation:

Where the FORESIGHT couples return having achieved good levels after the retest, the woman can be encouraged to drop the programme to:
2 FORESIGHT Vitamins;
2-3 FORESIGHT Minerals;
2 C-plus-Garlic.

If the magnesium, zinc, or manganese had been very low at the outset the appropriate supplement may still be given to hold the levels that have been achieved. It is then appropriate to suggest they try for a baby as soon as they wish. Often this will be achieved at the first ovulation thereafter.

If optimum levels have not been achieved by the first retest, the programme should be adjusted to fit the new levels and continued for as long as necessary.

In many cases the woman will become pregnant despite advice, when she is at the start of the supplement programme. The best option is for her to carry on with the full programme. Many healthy babies have been born with mothers taking the full FORESIGHT Programme throughout pregnancy. Every effort should be made to avoid deficiencies in this situation. And it needs to be understood that it is the deficiencies that pose a danger NOT the supplements.

Once pregnancy has been achieved we advise the woman to retest every three to four months throughout the pregnancy. This will give testing at around three months of pregnancy, and another at about seven months, which is ideal. We can them keep levels at the optimum throughout her pregnancy. This way our miscarriages are very, very rare and the babies are born in optimum health. Our recent research project showed 327 consecutive pregnancies without a miscarriage, a preterm birth or malformation. (Ward 1993)

Hair Chart 1

	Your results		Recommended Values	
Calcium	291		400	mg/kg
Magnesium	31		35	mg/kg
Potassium	60		75	mg/kg
Iron	20		30	mg/kg
Chromium	0.61		0.8	mg/kg
Cobalt	0.20		0.25	mg/kg
Copper	19		20	mg/kg
Manganese	1.13		1.5	mg/kg
Nickel	0.54		0.8	mg/kg
Selenium	1.08		2.25	mg/kg
Zinc	72		185	mg/kg

			Threshold values	
Aluminium	1.45		2.5	mg/kg
Cadmium	0.09		0.25	mg/kg
Mercury	0.07		0.4	mg/kg
Lead	1.22		1.0	mg/kg

Supplementation Programme

Supplement	Tablets	Time
FORESIGHT Vitamin Supplements	2	Mornings
FORESIGHT Mineral Supplements	3	Mornings
Dolomite 500	2	Mornings
Chromium GTF	1	Mornings
Selenium ACE	3	Lunchtimes
Zinc plus (B6, Mn)	3	6 pm
Manganese Plus	2	6 pm
Vitamin C + Garlic	4	Bedtime
Iron Orotate	2	Bedtime

Hair Chart 2

	Your results		Recommended Values
Calcium	237	400	mg/kg
Magnesium	37	35	mg/kg
Potassium	67	75	mg/kg
Iron	24	30	mg/kg
Chromium	1.14	0.8	mg/kg
Cobalt	0.36	0.25	mg/kg
Copper	30	20	mg/kg
Manganese	1.14	1.5	mg/kg
Nickel	0.58	0.8	mg/kg
Selenium	1.90	2.25	mg/kg
Zinc	121	185	mg/kg

			Threshold values
Aluminium	2.98	2.5	mg/kg
Cadmium	0.22	0.25	mg/kg
Mercury	0.17	0.4	mg/kg
Lead	5.20	1.0	mg/kg

Supplementation Programme

Supplement	Tablets	Time
FORESIGHT Vitamin Supplements	2	Mornings
FORESIGHT Mineral Supplements	3	Mornings
Calcium Orotate	2	Mornings
Zinc plus (B6, Mn)	3	6 pm
Manganese Plus	3	6 pm
Vitamin C + Garlic	8	Bedtime
HEP 194	2	Bedtime

Hair Chart 3

	Your results	Recommended Values	
Calcium	337	400	mg/kg
Magnesium	37	35	mg/kg
Potassium	80	75	mg/kg
Iron	32	30	mg/kg
Chromium	0.46	0.8	mg/kg
Cobalt	0.13	0.25	mg/kg
Copper	18	20	mg/kg
Manganese	0.84	1.5	mg/kg
Nickel	0.67	0.8	mg/kg
Selenium	1.41	2.25	mg/kg
Zinc	99	185	mg/kg
		Threshold values	
Aluminium	1.48	2.5	mg/kg
Cadmium	0.14	0.25	mg/kg
Mercury	0.13	0.4	mg/kg
Lead	4.78	1.0	mg/kg

Supplementation Programme

Supplement	Tablets	Time
FORESIGHT Vitamin Supplements	2	Mornings
FORESIGHT Mineral Supplements	3	Mornings
Dolomite 500	2	Mornings
Chromium GTF	3	Mornings
Cemac (vitamin B12)	3	Mornings
Manganese Plus	4	6 pm
Zinc plus (B6, Mn)	3	6 pm
Vitamin C + Garlic	8	Bedtime
Selenium ACE	3	Bedtime

Hair Chart 4

	Your results		Recommended Values
Calcium	306	400	mg/kg
Magnesium	29	35	mg/kg
Potassium	59	75	mg/kg
Iron	27	30	mg/kg
Chromium	0.61	0.8	mg/kg
Cobalt	0.26	0.25	mg/kg
Copper	13	20	mg/kg
Manganese	2.03	1.5	mg/kg
Nickel	0.81	0.8	mg/kg
Selenium	1.56	2.25	mg/kg
Zinc	117	185	mg/kg

			Threshold values
Aluminium	3.44	2.5	mg/kg
Cadmium	0.33	0.25	mg/kg
Mercury	0.13	0.4	mg/kg
Lead	4.95	1.0	mg/kg

Supplementation Programme

Supplement	Tablets	Time
FORESIGHT Vitamin Supplements	2	Mornings
FORESIGHT Mineral Supplements	3	Mornings
Calcium Orotate	2	Mornings
Magnesium Plus	2	Mornings
Zinc plus (B6, Mn)	3	6 pm
Efamol Marine	1	6 pm
Selenium ACE	3	Bedtime
Vitamin C + Garlic	8	Bedtime
HEP 194	1	Bedtime

117

Hair Chart 5

	Your results	Recommended Values	
Calcium	304	400	mg/kg
Magnesium	39	35	mg/kg
Potassium	100	75	mg/kg
Iron	29	30	mg/kg
Chromium	1.69	0.8	mg/kg
Cobalt	0.41	0.25	mg/kg
Copper	27	20	mg/kg
Manganese	1.44	1.5	mg/kg
Nickel	0.47	0.8	mg/kg
Selenium	1.23	2.25	mg/kg
Zinc	64	185	mg/kg

		Threshold values	
Aluminium	6.74	2.5	mg/kg
Cadmium	0.47	0.25	mg/kg
Mercury	0.21	0.4	mg/kg
Lead	8.73	1.0	mg/kg

Supplementation Programme

Supplement	Tablets	Time
FORESIGHT Vitamin Supplements	2	Mornings
FORESIGHT Mineral Supplements	4	Mornings
Zinc plus (B6, Mn)	3	6 pm
Efamol Marine	1	6 pm
Vitamin C + Garlic	8	Bedtime
HEP 194	1	Bedtime
Selenium (ACE)	3	Bedtime

Hair Chart 6

	Your results	Recommended Values	
Calcium	322	400	mg/kg
Magnesium	33	35	mg/kg
Potassium	71	75	mg/kg
Iron	31	30	mg/kg
Chromium	1.13	0.8	mg/kg
Cobalt	0.24	0.25	mg/kg
Copper	22	20	mg/kg
Manganese	1.28	1.5	mg/kg
Nickel	1.12	0.8	mg/kg
Selenium	2.21	2.25	mg/kg
Zinc	115	185	mg/kg

		Threshold values	
Aluminium	3.72	2.5	mg/kg
Cadmium	0.22	0.25	mg/kg
Mercury	0.22	0.4	mg/kg
Lead	4.91	1.0	mg/kg

Supplementation Programme

Supplement	Tablets	Time
FORESIGHT Vitamin Supplements	2	Mornings
FORESIGHT Mineral Supplements	3	Mornings
Calcium Orotate	2	Mornings
Magnesium Plus	1	Mornings
Zinc plus (B6, Mn)	3	6 pm
Efamol Marine	1	6 pm
Vitamin C + Garlic	8	Bedtime
HEP 194	1	Bedtime

Hair Chart 7

	Your results	Recommended Values	
Calcium	275	400	mg/kg
Magnesium	42	35	mg/kg
Potassium	71	75	mg/kg
Iron	36	30	mg/kg
Chromium	0.90	0.8	mg/kg
Cobalt	0.41	0.25	mg/kg
Copper	23	20	mg/kg
Manganese	0.74	1.5	mg/kg
Nickel	0.44	0.8	mg/kg
Selenium	3.12	2.25	mg/kg
Zinc	161	185	mg/kg
		Threshold values	
Aluminium	1.40	2.5	mg/kg
Cadmium	0.08	0.25	mg/kg
Mercury	0.06	0.4	mg/kg
Lead	1.22	1.0	mg/kg

Supplementation Programme

Supplement	Tablets	Time
FORESIGHT Vitamin Supplements	2	Mornings
FORESIGHT Mineral Supplements	3	Mornings
Calcium Orotate	3	Mornings
Zinc plus (B6, Mn)	2	6 pm
Manganese Plus	4	6 pm
Vitamin C + Garlic	3	Bedtime

Hair Chart 8

	Your results	Recommended Values	
Calcium	302	400	mg/kg
Magnesium	32	35	mg/kg
Potassium	71	75	mg/kg
Iron	22	30	mg/kg
Chromium	0.72	0.8	mg/kg
Cobalt	0.38	0.25	mg/kg
Copper	18	20	mg/kg
Manganese	1.14	1.5	mg/kg
Nickel	0.72	0.8	mg/kg
Selenium	1.72	2.25	mg/kg
Zinc	173	185	mg/kg

		Threshold values	
Aluminium	1.29	2.5	mg/kg
Cadmium	0.20	0.25	mg/kg
Mercury	0.17	0.4	mg/kg
Lead	1.48	1.0	mg/kg

Supplementation Programme

Supplement	Tablets	Time
FORESIGHT Vitamin Supplements	2	Mornings
FORESIGHT Mineral Supplements	3	Mornings
Calcium Orotate	2	Mornings
Magnesium Plus	2	Mornings
Selenium ACE	3	Lunchtimes
Zinc plus (B6, Mn)	1	6 pm
Manganese Plus	2	6 pm
Vitamin C + Garlic	3	Bedtime

Hair Chart 9

	Your results		Recommended Values	
Calcium	321	400	mg/kg
Magnesium	28	35	mg/kg
Potassium	52	75	mg/kg
Iron	28	30	mg/kg
Chromium	0.64	0.8	mg/kg
Cobalt	0.51	0.25	mg/kg
Copper	23	20	mg/kg
Manganese	1.30	1.5	mg/kg
Nickel	1.10	0.8	mg/kg
Selenium	2.00	2.25	mg/kg
Zinc	197	185	mg/kg

		Threshold values	
Aluminium	2.68	2.5	mg/kg
Cadmium	0.31	0.25	mg/kg
Mercury	0.29	0.4	mg/kg
Lead	9.99	1.0	mg/kg

Supplementation Programme

Supplement	Tablets	Time
FORESIGHT Vitamin Supplements	2	Mornings
FORESIGHT Mineral Supplements	3	Mornings
Calcium orotate	2	Mornings
Magnesium Plus	3	Mornings
Chromium GTF	2	Mornings
Zinc plus (B6, Mn)	2	6 pm
Efamol Marine	1	6 pm
Vitamin C + Garlic	8	Bedtime
Cantassium disc	1	Bedtime
HEP 194	2	Bedtime

Hair Chart 10

	Your results	Recommended Values	
Calcium	215	400	mg/kg
Magnesium	47	35	mg/kg
Potassium	61	75	mg/kg
Iron	33	30	mg/kg
Chromium	0.73	0.8	mg/kg
Cobalt	0.21	0.25	mg/kg
Copper	33	20	mg/kg
Manganese	0.32	1.5	mg/kg
Nickel	1.40	0.8	mg/kg
Selenium	0.72	2.25	mg/kg
Zinc	115	185	mg/kg

		Threshold values	
Aluminium	1.32	2.5	mg/kg
Cadmium	0.14	0.25	mg/kg
Mercury	0.08	0.4	mg/kg
Lead	3.72	1.0	mg/kg

Supplementation Programme

Supplement	Tablets	Time
FORESIGHT Vitamin Supplements	2	Mornings
FORESIGHT Mineral Supplements	3	Mornings
Calcium Orotate	3	Mornings
Chromium GTF	2	Mornings
Selenium ACE	3	Lunchtimes
Zinc plus (B6, Mn)	3	6 pm
Manganese Plus	4	6 pm
Vitamin C + Garlic	6	Bedtime

Hair Chart 11

	Your results		Recommended Values	
Calcium	417		400	mg/kg
Magnesium	35		35	mg/kg
Potassium	98		75	mg/kg
Iron	29		30	mg/kg
Chromium	0.64		0.8	mg/kg
Cobalt	0.22		0.25	mg/kg
Copper	19		20	mg/kg
Manganese	1.77		1.5	mg/kg
Nickel	1.29		0.8	mg/kg
Selenium	1.64		2.25	mg/kg
Zinc	131		185	mg/kg

			Threshold values	
Aluminium	4.72		2.5	mg/kg
Cadmium	0.13		0.25	mg/kg
Mercury	0.09		0.4	mg/kg
Lead	1.16		1.0	mg/kg

Supplementation Programme

Supplement	Tablets	Time
FORESIGHT Vitamin Supplements	2	Mornings
FORESIGHT Mineral Supplements	3	Mornings
Chromium GTF	2	Mornings
Zinc plus (B6, Mn)	3	6 pm
Efamol Marine	1	6 pm
Vitamin C + Garlic	6	Bedtime
Selenium (ACE)	3	Bedtime

Hair Chart 12

	Your results	Recommended Values	
Calcium	473	400	mg/kg
Magnesium	41	35	mg/kg
Potassium	98	75	mg/kg
Iron	25	30	mg/kg
Chromium	1.24	0.8	mg/kg
Cobalt	0.34	0.25	mg/kg
Copper	18	20	mg/kg
Manganese	1.34	1.5	mg/kg
Nickel	0.94	0.8	mg/kg
Selenium	1.20	2.25	mg/kg
Zinc	146	185	mg/kg

		Threshold values	
Aluminium	1.70	2.5	mg/kg
Cadmium	0.12	0.25	mg/kg
Mercury	0.10	0.4	mg/kg
Lead	2.30	1.0	mg/kg

Supplementation Programme

Supplement	Tablets	Time
FORESIGHT Vitamin Supplements	2	Mornings
FORESIGHT Mineral Supplements	3	Mornings
Zinc plus (B6, Mn)	2	6 pm
Efamol Marine	1	6 pm
Vitamin C + Garlic	3	Bedtime
Selenium ACE	4	Bedtime

Supplements used by FORESIGHT
A Rought Guide

Mineral	Hair Results	Appropriate Supplementation
Calcium	Below 370ppm	1 Calcium orotate
	Below 330ppm	2 Calcium orotate
	Below 270ppm	3 Calcium orotate
Magnesium	Below 32ppm	1 Magnesium plus
	Below 30ppm	2 Magnesium plus
	Below 26ppm	4 Magnesium plus
	Below 22ppm	6 Magnesium plus
Potassium	Below 50ppm	1 Cantassium disc
	Below 30ppm	2 Cantassium disc
Iron	Below 25ppm	1 Iron orotate
		or 1 FORESIGHT Iron Formula
	Below 19ppm	2 Iron orotate
		or 2 FORESIGHT Iron Formula

NB The FORESIGHT Iron Formula is appropriate if a small copper boost is required.

Copper	Below 12ppm	1/2 Copper orotate
	Below 8ppm	1 Copper orotate
Chromium	Below 0.6ppm	1 Chromium GTF
	Below 0.4ppm	2 Chromium GTF
Cobalt	Below 0.18ppm	1 Cemac
	Below 0.14ppm	2 Cemac
	Below 0.10ppm	3 Cemac
Manganese	Below 1.2ppm	1 Manganese plus
	Below 1.0ppm	2 Manganese plus
	Below 0.8ppm	3 Manganese plus
Nickel	Below 0.6ppm	Try Natural
		Dried Ocean Kelp 500mg
Selenium	Below 1.9ppm	1 Selenium ACE
	Below 1.7ppm	2 Selenium ACE
	Below 1.5ppm	3 Selenium ACE
Zinc	Below 175ppm	1 Zinc plus
	Below 160ppm	2 Zinc plus
	Below 140ppm	3 Zinc plus
	Below 110ppm	4 Zinc plus

Toxic Metals	Hair Results	Appropriate Supplementation
Aluminium	Above 2.5ppm	2 Vitamin C-plus-Garlic.
	Above 4.0ppm	4 Vitamin C-plus-Garlic.
	Above 6.0ppm	6 Vitamin C-plus-Garlic.
(Use also selenium and magnesium)		
Cadmium	Above 0.25ppm	2 Vitamin C-plus Garlic
	Above 0.4ppm	4 Vitamin C-plus Garlic
	Above 0.6ppm	6 Vitamin C-plus Garlic and 1 HEP 194
(Use also chromium)		
Lead	Above 1.5ppm	2 Vitamin C-plus Garlic
	Above 2.5ppm	4 Vitamin C-plus Garlic
	Above 3.5ppm	6 Vitamin C-plus Garlic
	Above 6ppm	8 Vitamin C-plus Garlic and 1 HEP 194

(Use also calcium, iron, manganese and zinc.)

Notes on the Previous Table

The programme needed to treat the highest level of toxin shown is appropriate. The quantities are not to be added. They should be used in conjunction with the appropriate balancing minerals as mentioned under supplementation, unless this mineral is already well in excess of the recommended value. Peas, beans, lentils, onions and garlic in the diet are said also to help.

All of the above tables must necessarily be adapted to individual circumstances, as no two charts are alike and the minerals are subject to interactions. Appropriate amounts may depend somewhat on a number of factors such as dietary and environmental changes which would have a positive effect. Mineral testing and interpretation of data, with suggested supplementation and cleansing programmes can be obtained from FORESIGHT. Details will be supplied on request.

Table 15:
Influence of Previous Reproductive Problems (mean female hair value,ug/g)

Function/Element	No History	Infertility	Miscarriage	Therapeutic Term.	Stillbirths	Small for date	Malform
age (y)	34	35	35	36	36	37	36
Ca	420	389	407	394	418	388	411
Mg	38	40	40	59	48	52	28
P	151	144	147	147	138	147	130
Na	175	133	143	160	181	157	167
K	92	61	61	54	70	71	40
Fe	26	26	26	27	27	27	26
Cu	28	28	28	30	23	27	19
Zn	170	159	169	169	163	151	141
Cr	0.73	0.71	0.72	0.69	0.81	0.76	0.8
Mn	1.56	1.52	1.46	1.4	1.7	1.25	1.2
Se	1.85	1.77	1.78	1.77	1.95	1.75	1.7
Ni	0.66	0.66	0.61	0.64	0.66	0.64	0.6
Co	0.24	0.21	0.2	0.22	0.26	0.21	0.2
Pb	3.8	3.5	3.8	3.8	4.3	3.5	6.9
Hg	0.43	0.41	0.42	0.43	0.32	0.39	0.48
Cd	0.19	0.18	0.17	0.21	0.15	0.16	0.38
As	0.12	0.15	0.12	0.12	0.1	0.11	0.11
Al	1.7	1.7	1.3	1.4	1.2	1.3	1.2

This chart reports the mean age (years) and mineral analysis for 367 females in terms of previous reproductive problem or non-problem (No History).

(Ward 1993)

Table 16 : Male Fertility Status and Hair Element (Calcium) Content (ug/g) – 367 males (Ward 1993)

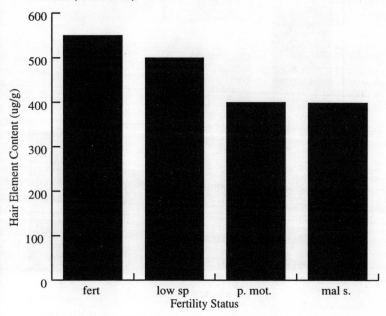

Table 17 : Male Fertility Status and Hair Element (Magnesium) Content (ug/g) –367 males (Ward 1993)

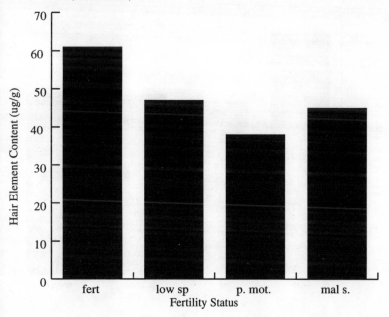

Table 18 : Male Fertility Status and Hair Element (Potassium) Content (ug/g) – 367 males (Ward 1993)

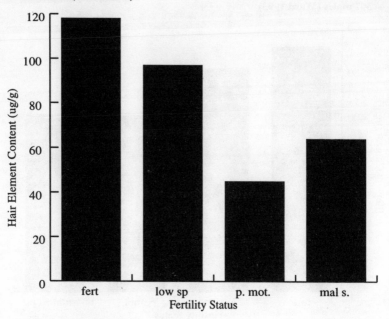

Table 19 : Male Fertility Status and Hair Element (Zinc) Content (ug/g) – 367 males (Ward 1993)

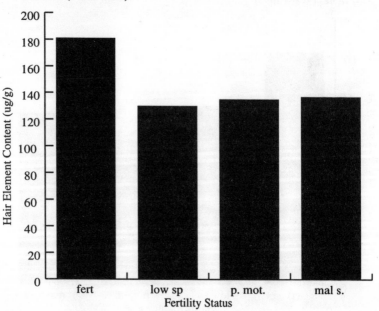

Table 20 : Male Fertility Status and Hair Element (Selenium) Content (ug/g) – 367 males (Ward 1993)

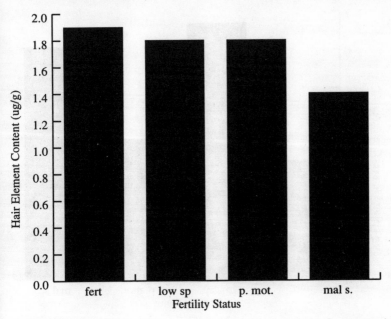

Table 21 : Male Fertility Status and Hair Element (Cadmium) Content (ug/g) – 367 males (Ward 1993)

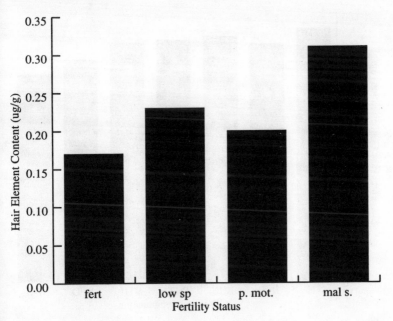

Table 22 : Male Fertility Status and Hair Element (Lead) Content (ug/g) – 367 males (Ward 1993)

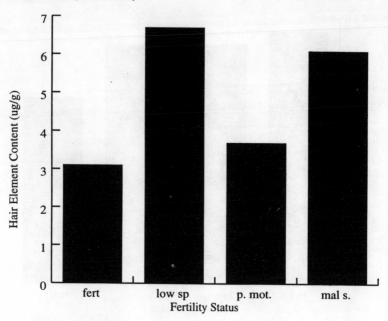

Table 23 : Hair Zn Content and Previous Pregnancy History – 367 females (Ward 1993)

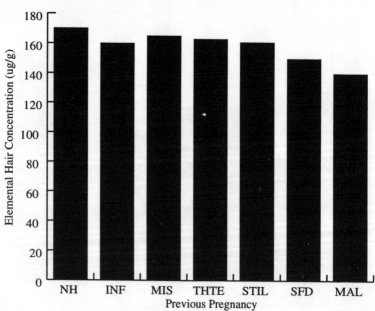

**Table 24 : Hair Pb Content and Previous Pregnancy History
– 367 females (Ward 1993)**

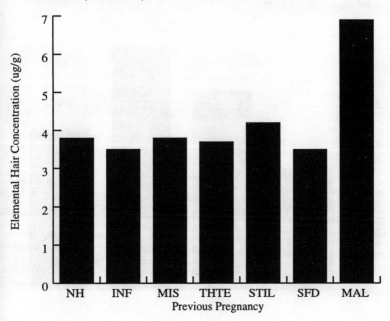

**Table 25 : Hair Cd Content and Previous Pregnancy History
– 367 females (Ward 1993)**

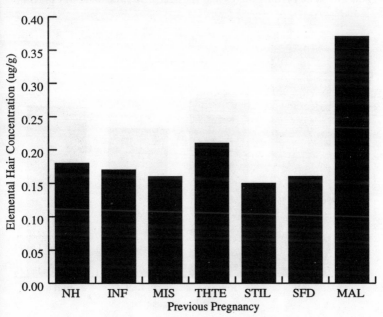

Table 26 : Hair Cd Concentration and Smoking Activity – 367 males (Ward 1993)

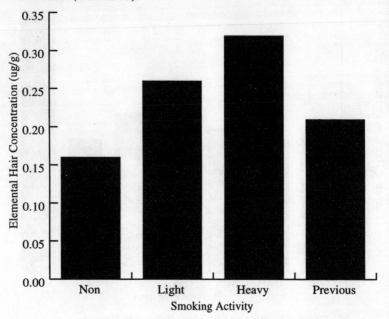

Table 27 : Male Fertility Status and Hair Element (Magnesium) Content (ug/g

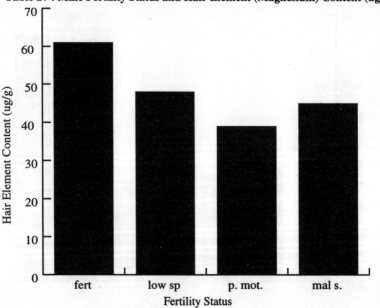

Hazards in the Workplace and Home

With women now forming a large part of the work-force and with greater recognition that occupational hazards can affect the male reproductive system it is recommended that the doctor takes fully into account at the preconception health care consultation any occupational health risk. The hazards are many, ranging from physical ones, such as radiation, VDUs, noise, light and heat, to chemical ones such as formaldehyde and benzene. (Franc 1981) The home is also not without its dangers, some brought in from the workplace, others from the environment, including the shopping bag.

Whatever the specific risk, however, there are two key points:
1 Prenatal exposure is more likely to produce toxic effects than adult exposure, so that although the pregnant woman may not seem to have health problems herself, her developing child may have.
2 Exposure to chemicals in the workplace can cause behavioural damage even without physical signs. One authority has suggested that "detection of behavioural deviations in children of mothers exposed to a hazardous substance while pregnant may be one of the most sensitive indicators of toxicity". (Spyker) (See radiation, heat and natural light, toxic metals, drugs and chemicals)

Noise

A Japanese study of 1,000 births linked lower birth weights with noise and lower levels of certain hormones believed to affect the fetal growth. (Polakoff 1984) It is not known what levels of maternal noise exposure may harm the fetus. Certainly since 1935 it has been known that effects of sound in general affect the fetus: Then it was found that a doorbell buzzer applied to the woman's abdomen in the last two months of pregnancy resulted in hyperactivity in the fetus and an increased fetal heart rate. (Ferreira 1969) Animals subjected to noise had higher rates of stillbirth, prematurity, malformations and abnormal birth weight than control animals. (Stuttaford 1988)

However, noise needs putting in context. Noise levels in the settings above were loud enough to cause undue stress to the body. The fetus is not growing in a noise-free environment: it is subjected to the noises in its mother's body, as well as those from her normal day-to-day activities. Pregnant women can be reassured that noise at general levels is part of the fetus's stimulation.

H eat

Numerous animal studies on a variety of species have confirmed the teratogenicity of heat. (Skreb 1963, Edwards 1967, Kilham 1976) An elevated maternal body temperature during early pregnancy disrupts mitotic processes in the developing embryo. (Webster 1984, Seller 1987, Shiota 1988)

In the man, heat can interfere with sperm production, since the testicles need to operate at a lower temperature than the rest of the body. Hours of sitting, such as happens with taxi and lorry drivers, travelling salesmen and business executives may result in excess scrotal heat. (Andrews 1984) Skin-tight underwear or frequent hot baths can have a similar effect. (Teymor 1978)

The teratogenic effects of hyperthermia in the woman are more controversial, although there is good evidence to suggest they exist. Hyperthermia tends to stop the division of cells and very high temperatures may even kill cells. (Teymor 1978) In the fetus, cell division is basic to growth so stopping it can have devastating consequences. Both brain size and function have been affected. Some research suggests that in cases of fever, the high temperature alone can cause damage. One study of brain damaged children revealed that their mothers had taken prolonged saunas. (Smith 1979) An American study of neural tube defect etiology found that "hot-bath use increased the risk of spina bifida approximately 31-fold." (Sandford 1992) A further study has suggested a strong association between febrile illness and anencephalus. (Shiota 1982)

Some of the scepticism has arisen from the low rate of anencephalus among the Finns, where sauna bathing is common.(Leck 1978) However, it would seem that short sauna, six to ten minutes long, such as practised by the Finns, may be safe. One study raised an additional concern about the potential effects of hot baths when it found that most women did not experience discomfort or they leave the spa bath before their core temperature had reached 39 degrees centigrade. (Ridge 1990)

RECOMMENDATIONS: It is advisable that men should wear clothing which allows the scrotum to keep cooler than the rest of the body and avoid prolonged soaking in the hot bath as this may temporarily diminish the mobility of the sperm, though it is not known if this might be injurious should pregnancy ensue.

Women who are pregnant, or who think/hope they may be pregnant, are advised to avoid hot baths or showers. Prolonged saunas are best avoided during the first three to five months of pregnancy. Short saunas, six to ten minutes long, as taken by the Finns, seem safe. However, the woman may prefer to avoid saunas altogether during pregnancy. Electric blankets should not be used. Where there is a febrile illness every effort should be made to lower the temperature as soon as possible.

Intestinal Infestation
by Dr Belinda Dawes

Parasites

Intestinal parasites are a common and unsuspected cause of chronic disease. They are a common cause of problems such as diarrhoea, constipation and bloating, intestinal malabsorption, food intolerance, chronic fatigue, fever and immunological dysfunction.

The most common parasites encountered in the United States, the United Kingdom and Australia are protozoa (one-celled animals). Two of these are of such significance that all doctors should be familiar with them: Giardia lamblia and Entamoeba histolytica. Also of importance are Endolimax Nana and Blastocystis hominus.

Parasite infection is transmitted through contaminated food and water and sometimes by sexual intercourse. People who live together may get parasites from each other by sharing the same bathroom or by preparing food for each other. Some parasites are transmitted by insect bites or contact with contaminated soil. Animals, including domestic pets, are subject to Giardia infection.

Giardia contaminates streams, rivers and lakes in mountainous regions. It can also contaminate wells and municipal water supplies. Giardia lives in the upper small intestine where the inflammation it produces can cause severe pain, bloating, gas, diarrhoea, food intolerance, indigestion, malabsorption and loss of enzymes. Chronic infections may produce constipation, fatigue and weight loss. Chronic giardiasis may cause illness misdiagnosed as chronic Epstein-Barr virus infection. Giardia also has an affinity for candida albicans and may contribute to intestinal candidiasis, and chronic candida infection predisposes to giardiasis. The incidence in the United States of America is 7.5 per cent

Entamoeba histolytica is generally considered a tropical parasite but may be found anywhere in the world. The incidence in the United States of America is 3%. The great increase in foreign travel and the immigration of people from areas with high E. histolytica prevalence have made the parasite almost as common as Giardia lamblia in the New York metropolis area. E. histolytica inhabits the large intestine. As with Giardia, infections may produce no symptoms whatsoever. Severe infection can cause amebic dysentery, a condition which, when chronic, mimics the disease ulcerative colitis. Such infection can also spread to the liver and other organs. Milder infections, which are more common, can cause diarrhoea and/or constipation, pain, bloating, food intolerance, immune suppression, fatigue, allergic reactions and reactive inflammation of joints and muscles. E histolytica infection is considered to be a possible predisposing factor for the development for AIDS from HIV, due to the immune suppression.

Diagnosis

Most physicians rely in stool analysis to search for intestinal parasites. However, because Giardia is an upper intestinal parasite, stool examination is a very poor technique for tracing it. The combination of rectal swab for obtaining the specimen and fluorescent microscopy for examining the specimens yields results that are far superior to the standard evaluation. The mucus obtained from the rectal swab is mixed with special stains and examined under the microscope for the presence of parasites, yeasts and abnormal bacteria. The stains used in this technique are:

1 Iodine stain for parasites and parasite eggs.

2 A special trichome stain to confirm results on the iodine stain.

3 A monoclonal antibody fluorescent stain for Giardia lamblia.

4 A monoclonal antibody fluorescent stain for Cryptosporidum.

5 A flourescent stain for yeasts and a culture for yeast.

6 Acid fast and fluorescent stains for Campylobacter.

7 A fluorescent stain for enteropathogenic E. coli.

8 A fluorescent stain for antibodies to disease producing stains of the parasite Entamoeba histolytica.

Therapy

Successful therapy of chronic protoal infection can be use of the herbal preparation Artmieisa Annua. The active ingredient in artemiesia, a substance called quing hsao, has been shown to kill malaria organisms that are resistant to all other known drugs. Chronic infection needs to be treated for several weeks or months to produce complete resolution. There are many forms of artemesia available, some poisonous. Artmieisa Annua is contra indicated during pregnancy, so treatment must be completed prior to conception.

A pregnant woman with a parasite infection will suffer malabsorption and fatigue, thereby affecting both mother and fetus. More importantly, prescription drugs used to treat parasites cannot be used during pregnancy. It is therefore essential to test for parasitic infection before pregnancy occurs in all women where an index gives a suspicion that parasites exist.

It is also important to consider the transmission of parasitic infection to a child if parents remain untreated. Small babies are far more seriously affected by diarrhoea than adults and it can be life-threatening. Any positive outcome should result in family members being tested.

Minerals

Calcium

is needed for the formation of strong bones and teeth, and for controlling blood clotting mechanisms and proper nerve and muscle function. Other functions include assisting in muscle growth, maintaining blood balance and acting as a catalyst in enzyme reactions It may help to protect against allergies, viruses and tooth decay.   In pregnancy, calcium is vital for the growth of the fetus and the well being of the mother. Davis recommends giving it, in conjunction with vitamin D, during labour to ease pain. It can ease leg cramps. Low levels are associated with low birth weight and low scores on developmental tests. Premature babies tend to have low levels. Calcium is lost from the bones during bed rest and also on high protein diets. People affected will need to supplement the diet and to choose foods with high levels. Lack of calcium can cause rickets, back pain, osteoporosis, osteomalacia, irritability, nervousness, tension, uneven heart beat, indigestion, stomach cramps and spasms, constipation, pre-menstrual tension and cramping of the uterus. (Davies 1954, Davies 1974, Pitkin 1975, Nutrition Search Inc 1979, Passwater 1983)

Sources: Kelp, cheese, carob, bone broth, green vegetables, brazil nuts, whole raw milk (pasteurisation reduces calcium availability), dolomite, brewer's yeast, yoghurt.

Foods containing oxalic acid (sesame seed hulls, rhubarb, spinach) and phytic acid (soda and unleavened bread) can reduce availability.

It is best taken with vitamins A, C, D, essential fatty acids (EFA), iron, magnesium, phosphorus. (Nutrition Search Inc 1979)

Chromium

is needed for the regulation of the glucose tolerance factor, in combination with nicotinic acid and some proteins. Glucose is required for every bodily function. Chromium is also necessary for the synthesis of fatty acids and cholesterol. A deficiency may be linked with heart disease. (Passwater 1983)

Chromium is not easily absorbed, though it is readily removed from the body. Even a small deficiency will be serious.

Sources: Brewer's yeast, black pepper, liver, whole grains, wheat germ, vegetables, butter, beer, molasses.

Cobalt

is an essential part of vitamin B12. There is a possible relationship between cobalt and iodine. It is necessary in B12 for the normal functioning of all cells, but especially red blood cells, and has been used in the treatment of pernicious anaemia. However, there are serious toxic side effects so its role is of limited value. It activates some enzymes. Deficiency is associated with pernicious anaemia, and maybe with slow growth and goitre. (Underwood 1977, Nutrition Search Inc 1979)

Sources: Although it is said that cobalt can only be taken in humans in the form of vitamin B12, Underwood points out that organ meat and muscle meats each contain more than can be accounted for as B12. Green leafy vegetables are a good source if the soil was rich, but others include meats, brewer's yeast, seafood, nuts, fruits and whole grains.

Cobalt is more effective when taken with copper, iron and zinc. (Nutrition Search Inc 1979)

Copper

aids the development of the brain, bones, nerves and connective tissue. It is involved in many enzyme systems, and is essential in the production of RNA.

Deficiency can cause porous bones, loss of hair, demyelination, heart damage and anaemia.

In the fetus of a number of animals, copper deficiency can result in depressed growth, depigmentation, anaemia, fine fragile bones, ataxia, small brain and perinatal mortality. In rats, infertility has been noted. Skeletal and cardiovascular defects, central nervous system disorders, and "steely wool" hair (failure of melanin formation) have also been reported. (Nutrition Search Inc 1979, Passwater 1983, Underwood 1977)

Copper deficiency is rare however, and copper in excess can be toxic. (See toxic metals)

Sources: Shellfish, brazil nuts, organ meats, dried legumes, dried stone fruits and green vegetables

It is best taken with cobalt, iron and zinc. (Nutrition Search Inc 1979)

Iodine

is necessary for the formation of thyroxine and triiodothyronine. Thyroxine is necessary for growth, mental and physical development and the maintenance of health. Most people are aware that too little iodine can cause goitres, but deficiency is also associated with fatigue, lethargy, susceptibility to cold, loss of interest in sex, slow development of sex organs, anorexia, slow pulse, low blood pressure, rapid weight gain, high blood cholesterol, death from heart disease and cancer of the thyroid.

Deficiency in the pregnancy can result in cretinism in children, a congenital disease with mental and physical retardation. If iodine is given soon after birth, many of the symptoms are reversible. (Passwater 1983, Nutition search Inc 1979, Davis 1974, Pharoach 1971)

Sources: include water, iodised salt, watercress, onions, kelp, shellfish, mushrooms and dark, leafy vegetables if they are grown on soil rich in iodine.

Too much iodine can also have serious consequences for health. (Underwood 1977, Nutrition Search Inc 1979)

Iron

is needed to make haemoglobin, the substance in red blood cells, which carries oxygen to the muscles. It helps in protein digestion and also in respiratory function

Needs in pregnancy increase because the number of red blood cells increase by 30 per cent. Since most women do not have a large enough store before pregnancy, the small amounts of iron in the diet may not be sufficient, so many women are given supplements. This can be quite unsatisfactory if other nutrients are not also given, since iron is not absorbed well without vitamin C and needs to work with other vitamins and minerals. Iron given alone can also cause loss of other essential minerals, such as zinc, manganese, chromium, selenium and cobalt.

Shortage of iron can lead to weakness, excessive fatigue, depression, headache, pallor, lack of appetite, mental confusion and poor memory. Iron deficient people will absorb two to three times more lead than non-deficient people. Deficiency is not so common in men, but it does occur in children, particularly if they are eating a diet which includes white flour and white sugar.

In the fetus, iron deficiency can cause eye defects, slow growth, bone defects, brain defects and neonatal mortality. (Nutrition Search Inc 1979, Pitkin 1972, Gibbs 1980, Lesser 1980, Passwater 1983, Davis 1974, Watson 1980, Oberleas 1972)

Sources: Organ meats, liver, kelp, brewer's yeast, molasses, wheat germ, almonds, parsley, egg yolk, lean meats, whole grains, vegetables. The iron of egg yolk is poorly absorbed unless taken with a food containing vitamin C. Thus, a glass of fresh orange juice with an egg is a good source of iron. (Nutrition Search Inc 1979)

Blood donors of both sexes are at risk of iron deficiency, so giving blood when planning a pregnancy is not advisable.

The usual test for iron is using blood. However, since the body will draw from its stores in the tissues and bones to maintain the amount in circulation, blood is not the best way of checking levels. For this reason, some doctors prefer to use hair samples as well.

Magnesium

is needed for the production and transfer of energy, muscle contraction, proper nerve function, protein synthesis and the functioning of many enzymes.

Deficiencies cause involuntary muscle movements, such as spasms and twitching, convulsions, insomnia, irregular heart beat, leg and foot cramps, bedwetting and depression. Pregnancy aggravates any deficiency. A deficiency is said to contribute to painful uterine contractions at the end of pregnancy. It may also be associated with miscarriage or premature birth. Rats fed low magnesium diets give birth to smaller pups with a higher rate of congenital deformities. They also develop calcium deposits and other abnormalities in heart cells. Women with low levels tend to abort more or have low birth weight babies. (Pfeiffer 1978, Davis 1974, Hurley 1976, Spatling 1988). Magnesium deficiency is very common.

Sources: Nuts, kelp, green vegetables, seafood, eggs, milk, whole grains, dolomite.

Magnesium is best taken with Vitamins B6, C, D, calcium, phosphorus, protein. (Nutrition Search Inc 1979)

Manganese

is needed for numerous enzyme reactions, bone growth and development, lipid metabolism and nerve function. It is necessary in the formation of thyroxine and in blood clotting. It may contribute to a mother's maternal instincts and love, through its role in certain enzymes. Although its function in reproduction is not understood, there is no doubt that a deficiency can affect fetal development. In a study of hair levels of manganese, babies with congenital malformations had significantly lower levels of manganese than babies without malformations.(Saner 1985) There were also similarly significant differences in the mineral levels of the mother's hair.

In rats it has been shown that in the least severe stage there is an increase in the number of offspring born with ataxia. In the second, more serious stage, the young are born dead or die shortly after birth, while in the third, most serious stage, the parent animal will not mate and sterility occurs. This is also seen in hens. In the male rat and rabbit with severe deficiency there is sterility, and also absence of sex drive, associated with degeneration of the seminal tubes and lack of spermatozoa. In the young there may be faulty cartilage and bone matrix formation and heart and neural function problems. Animals from mothers who are deficient show difficulty with behavioural tasks. (Williams 1973, Pfeiffer 1978, Underwood 1977, Oberleas 1972, Saner 1985)

Sources: Nuts, whole grains, seeds, leafy green vegetables, brewer's yeast, egg, liver, parsley, thyme, cloves, ginger, tea (see drugs).
    It is best taken with vitamin B1, E, calcium, phosphorus. (Nutrition Search Inc 1979)
    Uptake of manganese is inhibited by choline deficiency. (see Vitamins)

Nickel
is found in high concentrations of RNA and DNA and in all tissues and fluids. Most of the work on it has been focused on animals. It is needed for the action in the enzyme urease. In studies, deficiencies have been linked with reproductive failures and growth problems. In the rat, it is associated with the metabolism of copper and manganese. It may have a role in hormonal control and as an enzyme cofactor. High levels are found in the blood of patients who have suffered heart attacks. It is thought that the damaged heart muscles release the nickel. Levels are decreased in those with cirrhosis of the liver, or chronic uraemia. Deficiency is claimed to have a negative influence on growth and life expectancy and to impair iron metabolism.(Underwood 1977, Pfeiffer 1975, Neilson 1984a and b, Anke Undated, Pfeiffer 1978, Spears 1984)

Sources : Soya beans, dry beans, lentils, nuts, buckwheat, grains, vegetables and kelp supplements.

Sources not recommended: It is also found in hydrogenated vegetable oils, such as corn, as it is used as a catalyst in the processing. (Nutrition Search Inc 1979) Too much nickel can also have serious health risks. (Pfeiffer 1978)

Phosphorus
is the second most abundant mineral in the body, being found in every cell. As it functions with calcium, both being the main constituents of bone, it is important that its balance with calcium is maintained. It plays a part in almost every chemical reaction in the body, in the utilisation of carbohydrates, proteins and fats, in muscle and nerve function, digestion, kidney function and proper skeletal growth. It is found in important substances called phospholipids, which

break up and transport the fatty acids. Among their many functions are the promotion and the secretion of glandular hormones.

Deficiency is rare, since it is found in artificial fertilisers. It is also a common ingredient in many food additives and soft drinks. The right way to ensure balancing it with calcium and other minerals is to obtain it from whole foods. (Pfeiffer 1978, Nutrition Search Inc 1979, Davis 1974)

Sources: Brewer's yeast, whole grains, bread, cereals, meat, fish, poultry, eggs, seeds, nuts.

Phosphorus is best taken with vitamins A, D, EFA, calcium, iron, manganese and protein. (Nutriton Search Inc 1979)

Potassium

is needed to regulate blood pH, to acidify urine and for proper nerve and muscle functioning. It is involved in the utilisation of enzymes. It may be involved in bone calcification. Together with sodium, it maintains the fluid balance in the body and may help in the transportation of nutrients into the cells. It is necessary for growth.

A deficiency causes nervous irritability, insomnia, oedema, headaches, irregular heart beat, bone and joint pain, constipation, cramping of muscles, weakness and fatigue. It may be linked to poor sperm motility. In the embryo it may cause abnormalities in the kidneys. Deficiency may result from too much sodium chloride (salt), too little fruit and vegetables, some diseases and some medical treatments. Potassium deficiency may be related to poor sperm motility. Potassium chloride has been used successfully in the treatment of children's colic, and diarrhoea in adults as well as children. (Passwater 1983, Nutrition Search Inc 1979, Hurley 1976)

Sources: Brewer's yeast, wheat germ, whole grains, vegetables, fruits, nuts.

Potassium is best taken with Vitamin B6 and sodium. (Nutrition Search Inc 1979)

Selenium

like Vitamin E with which it is associated in some functions, is a powerful anti-oxidant which helps to prevent chromosomal damage in tissue culture. Such damage is associated with birth defects and cancers. It is a vital part of an important enzyme which helps the body to fight infections. In animals and chickens, deficiencies are associated with slow growth, cataracts, infertility, loss of hair and feathers, degeneration, nutritional muscular dystrophy, swelling and haemorrhages, pancreatic atrophy and liver necrosis. In human cell culture it is required for growth. Selenium will combine with toxic metals, such as cadmium, so it is useful for detoxification. It may be important in preventing cot deaths. In the USA about a quarter of the babies who die each year are found to be deficient in selenium and/or Vitamin E. Most of them are bottle fed. (Pfeiffer 1978, Underwood 1977)

Sources: Butter, smoked herring, wheat germ, brazil nuts, brewer's yeast, whole grains, garlic and liver. For the baby, human milk is an excellent source.

Selenium can also be toxic, though. FORESIGHT practitioners have found excesses in people who use selenium containing anti-dandruff shampoos in the bath, and then soak in the water. It is possible that some Xerox copying machines can also produce selenium in the atmosphere.

Selenium is more effective when taken with Vitamin E. (Nutrition Search Inc 1979)

Silicon

is crucial in the formation of connective tissues, bones, the placenta, arteries and skin, keeping it impermeable. It has been found to be essential for growth and skeletal development in rats and chicks. (Underwood 1977, Passwater 1973)

Sources: Whole grains, wholemeal bread, alfalfa, vegetables, especially the skins, pectin and hard water.

Vanadium

is present in most tissues in the body and is rapidly excreted into urine. It is thought to exert some influence on lipid metabolism by inhibiting cholesterol formation. It is part of the natural circulatory regulating system. Raised levels are possibly involved in the aetiology of manic depressive psychosis. Deficiency in animals results in impaired bone development, reduced growth, and disturbance of blood metabolism, decreased reproduction and increased perinatal mortality, and reduced fertility in subsequent generations. (Underwood 1977, Naylor 1984, Nielson 1984)

Sources: Buckwheat, parsley, Soya beans, eggs, sunflower seed oil, olive oil, olives, oats, rice, green beans, vegetables.

Zinc

is needed for health and maintenance of hormone levels, bones, muscles and sperm. It is important in healing. It is needed for the functioning of at least 200 enzymes. It is an important component of semen. It is necessary to stabilise RNA. It is needed in Vitamin A metabolism. It is essential for brain development and function. Caldwell and Oberleas have shown in rats that "even a mild zinc deficiency has a potential influence on behaviour potential despite an apparently adequate protein level in the diet."

In the male, zinc can increase the size of the penis and testes in growing boys. It also increases sperm motility and helps to prevent impotence.

Lack of zinc is associated with a loss of the senses of taste and smell, both of which affect appetite and anorexia. In animals, eye problems, high rates of miscarriage (resorption), brain malformation, cleft palate, cleft lip, club feet, stillbirth and urinary-genital abnormalities have been found. Low levels in maternal rats have been associated with learning problems and behavioural problems in their offspring. With all the concern about a general weakening of the immune system, it is worrying to note that in an experiment with mice, damage occurred to the immune system of offspring whose mothers were zinc deficient. The damage persisted even when supplements of zinc were given.

Low zinc status in the mother is a factor in infertility, and low birth weight. Low plasma levels at mid pregnancy have been associated with more complications of delivery and a higher incidence of malformations. Deficiencies have been found in children with learning disabilities, especially dyslexia. Low levels were found in the hair of children suffering from anorexia, poor growth and hypogeusia (loss of taste). (Sandstead 1984, Pfeiffer 1978, Crosby 1977, Crawford 1975, Caldwell 1969, Bryce-smith 1986, Hurley 1969, Jameson 1984, Ward 1987, Lazebnik 1988, Grant 1985, Hambidge 1972, Nutrition Search Inc 1979)

Sources: Oysters, whole grains, meat, brewer's yeast. wheat germ, fruit, vegetables, nuts, offal, fish, poultry and shellfish.

Zinc is best taken with Vitamin A, calcium, copper and phosphorus. (Nutrition Search Inc 1979)

Multi-element studies

Multi-element studies are few. The latest work has been the FORESIGHT research conducted at the University of Surrey. This revealed that the mineral status of the male is closely linked to his reproductive ability. Of special importance in relation to problems with conception were inadequate levels of calcium, potassium, zinc, chromium and possibly iron and manganese. There were also problems associated with raised levels of lead, cadmium, aluminium, and possibly mercury. Sperm problems were associated with lower levels of zinc and possibly selenium, especially for malformed sperm, and high levels of lead and cadmium. Poor motility was linked with low levels of calcium, magnesium and potassium.

Studying the previous reproductive history in females, there were significant differences between those who had had normal births and those showing previous problems related to pregnancy, including infertility, miscarriage, therapeutic terminations, stillbirths, small for date or low birth weight and malformations. The data demonstrated that, in general, those having malformed babies or stillbirths showed high levels of toxic metals and low levels of essential elements. Ward found that those women with no previous problems had higher zinc levels than those with previous problems. (Ward 1993)

Natural Family Planning (NFP)

Throughout history people have linked times in the cycle with fertility – not always the right times! Misunderstandings have led to loss of confidence in various methods, especially the rhythm method (calendar method), widely recommended in the past by the Roman Catholic Church. The Church now recommends Natural Family Planning (NFP) as advocated here. NFP is not a rhythm method and should never be confused with it. Modern NFP is derived from the latest knowledge about the monthly cycle, the same knowledge on which the contraceptive pill was developed, though there the similarity with the pill ends!

Pregnancy can only occur when an active sperm meets an egg that is ready to be fertilised. Since the egg can only survive for up to 24 hours and the sperm can survive for three to six days, it follows that pregnancy can only happen if intercourse takes place during the vulnerable seven days in each monthly cycle. Natural family planning methods aim to identify these days so that a couple can either take measures to avoid pregnancy or use the knowledge to conceive.

The advantages of NFP have been listed by Dr Anna Flynn, a leading expert. They include:

No known side effects;

More awareness of fertility, which helps to promote a more responsible attitude to family planning and sometimes a better relationship between partners;

A morally acceptable and viable method for those for whom abstinence but not other methods are suitable;

Personal control over fertility;

Once taught, there is no need for follow-up or further expenses.

It can help achieve pregnancy, (when this is the desired aim). (Flynn 1985)

Like every other method there are disadvantages, including a failure rate which may be as low as one per cent or up to twenty to thirty per cent, depending on which study is quoted. Flynn identifies three important factors which contribute to success or failure:

1 Motivation

More success is reported among users who want to limit their families than among those who are spacing pregnancies or delaying them.

2 Efficient teaching

Success depends on identifying the fertile period and this is best taught, ideally to both partners, by competent teachers. For those unable to see a teacher a video is available from the Fertility Trust but it is not yet known how successful it is in teaching the method effectively. However, it has been written by Dr Flynn and couples following it are likely to be well-motivated.

3 Characteristics of the woman

Some find it difficult to identify the various types of mucus, though a WHO study of 896 women in five countries and with varied backgrounds, including illiteracy, found that 97 per cent could do so correctly. (WHO 1981)

4 If abstinence is the option, it may be hard at a time when, for many, libido is high.

A combination of high motivation and good teaching in the largest study undertaken of NFP was shown to produce a failure rate of only 0.2 per cent pregnancies per 100 women, a rate which compares with that of the combined contraceptive pill – without the risks of the pill! (Rydar 1993) Indeed, data accumulating from around the world is confirming that the effectiveness of NFP is as good as that of other methods of family planning.

Central to NFP is the recognition of fertile period. There are three main ways of identifying the fertile days:

1 Checking the mucus.

2 Checking the cervix.

3 The temperature method.

In practice, the couple should be advised to use at least 1 and 2 together, or preferably all three to obtain maximum reliability.

Checking the mucus

This method (and checking the cervix) can tell when ovulation is about to happen. It is important to be able to calculate in advance when this will take place since sperm can survive in the vagina for up to five days around the time of ovulation. At other times they die within a few hours as they cannot live in the usually acidic environment of the vagina.

Early in the cycle several eggs begin to ripen in the ovary, producing increasing amounts of oestrogen, the female sex hormone. Oestrogen causes the production of mucus from the cervix, mucus which helps the sperm to survive in the vagina, and to travel to meet the egg when it is released at ovulation. After menstruation, the vagina and vuvla feel dry because little mucus is being released. The level of oestrogen is low, and the mucus is cloudy, thick, sticky, lethal to sperm and so is able to stop the sperm from entering the womb. However, as the level of oestrogen rises, the mucus becomes more watery, clear, and, like egg-white, slippery and stretchy. The vagina and vulva feel moist or wet and the vagina becomes alkaline, a condition suitable for the sperm's survival. Sometimes mid-cycle bleeding occurs and the mucus is pinkish. The last day of fertile mucus is called "Peak Day" as it is the day when ovulation is most likely to occur. After ovulation the mucus dries up again to form a plug in the cervix which stops any sperm getting through in case there has been a fertilisation. The first three days after Peak Day are regarded as fertile days, to allow for the release, life and death of the egg and the complete reforming of the mucus plug. The rest of the cycle is infertile. It is easy to observe the mucus by wiping the vulva with toilet tissue. The woman should also record her subjective feelings of wetness or dryness, ideally noting them on a chart on which she records her temperature. (See below, The Temperature Method)

Checking the cervix
Not only does the mucus change throughout the cycle, so does the state of the cervix, the changes correlating to those of the mucus. When the ovum is ready to be fertilised the os opens to help the sperm meet the ovum. When the ovum is not ready to be fertilised, the os closes to stop the sperm entering the womb. These changes can be felt, though in a woman who has had a baby, the os may never fully close.

In the infertile phase the cervix is low in the vagina, the os is closed and there is a firm, dry, maybe gritty feel. As the cycle moves into its fertile phase, the cervix changes, becoming softer and sticky, with the mucus forming. In the fertile phase it is high in the vagina, soft, slippery, rubbery, with the os fully opened. After the fertile phase it reverts to its low, firm state.

The temperature method
This depends on the rise and fall in temperature that naturally occurs throughout the cycle, as the body warms up to act as a natural incubator if fertilisation occurs. When the ovum is released the woman's temperature may drop very slightly, which is noticeable using a special thermometer. Immediately afterwards, because of the release of progesterone, the temperature of the body at complete rest rises between 0.2-0.4 degrees centigrade, staying at the higher level until menstruation. When it has been at the higher level for three days, it is unlikely that the ovum will be fertilised by any sperm which may still be present.

To use this method the woman should be advised to take her temperature with a fertility thermometer on waking, before doing anything, and to record the result on a fertility chart. She should record any factor that could have affected the reading, such as: lack of sleep, shock, travel or shift work, to mention but a few. Drugs such as aspirin can lower body temperature, confusing the chart. A high temperature for more than 20 days may mean a pregnancy.

The disadvantage of the method is that it cannot tell when ovulation is going to occur and when the fertile phase begins. It is therefore essential that it is used in conjunction with the mucus method.

If a woman has a regular cycle however ovulation will occur on the same day each month, so can be predicted with accuracy.

Natural Light
(This section is partly based on a talk by Dr Damien Downing on "Natural Light and Ovulation Patterns" given in December 1991)

In 1909 Otto Marburg made the observation that the pineal gland might have an antigonadatrophin effect. Not only has this been proven, the mechanism is also understood.

The pineal gland does not alter much in size throughout life, nor does the output of its principle hormone, melatonin, vary much. As well as producing drowsiness and encouraging sleep, and a possible role in Seasonal Affective Disorder, this hormone has a clear effect on fertility in a large number of animals. (Rosenthal 1985) It is the device whereby those mammals that have an oestrous cycle trigger fertility at certain times of the year in order to take advantages of seasons. The way this operates varies depending on the length of gestation of the animal concerned. For example, the larger animals such as cows and sheep with a gestation lasting several months tend to come into season in autumn, triggered by reducing day length and consequent rising melatonin levels. This leads to pregnancy being carried throughout the winter, and the offspring being born in the spring, with the whole of summer in which to grow before being exposed to the risks of winter. In smaller animals, such as a number of rodents, oestrous is triggered by increasing day length and, therefore, falling levels of melatonin levels. Gestation thus starts in the spring and finishes in early summer, with the same benefits. Research has shown that mice kept in artificial light conditions had young who died prematurely or had very small litters, suggesting the need to research the role of light further. (Ott 1985)

Ultra violet
The ultra violet part of the radiation known as sunlight is the most biologically active. Ultra violet wavelengths can kill bacteria, and are used by some water suppliers in their purification processes. Ultra violet radiation has also been provided by law to miners in Russia to help remove dust from their lungs. (Kime 1980)

154

Ultra violet rays can be UV-A or UV-B type. The UV-B type are the stronger and cause sunburn, although one expert has said that the weaker UV-A does the same damage, and may be even worse. His reasoning is that to tan one has to have the same overall exposure, so that with UV-A one will need to expose oneself for longer. However, the UV-A penetrated deeper than UV-B and may cause damage to collagen, blood vessels and elastic tissues. UV-B may therefore be safer because UV-A lulls one into a false sense of security. Also, once exposed to UV-A, the body is more suspectible to the ageing and carcinogenic effects of UV-B radiation. (McCarthy 1988)

There is now much discussion about exposure to the sun and skin cancer. To induce skin cancer in animals it is necessary to give larger-than normal doses of ultra violet light so that burning occurs.(Kime 1980) There seems to be a direct relationship between the amount of free radicals formed in the skin when it is exposed to sunlight and the tendency for the skin to burn. Stop the free radicals forming and you considerably reduce the sunburning. Another factor that may be significant is cholesterol, which may be changed into a number of products when the ultra violet rays strike the skin, one of which, cholesterol alphaoxide, can act as a free radical and cause cancer. Oils and fats applied to the skin, or sunbathing creams, may also stimulate cancer formation. (Kime 1980) Free radical formation can be inhibited by certain nutrients in the diet, including Vitamins A, C, and E.

Nutrition – its vital role in pregnancy

The concept of biochemical individuality
In 1956 Dr Roger Williams, an American Biochemist found that every individual is biochemically different. This means that everyone has needs for levels of nutrients that are individual to them alone, especially in respect of vitamins, minerals and amino acids. Research has shown, for example, that some individuals may need many times the recommended levels of a vitamin or mineral if they are to remain healthy. (Williams 1956) In certain conditions, such as pregnancy, requirements will alter.

The importance of food before pregnancy
Although it is essential to eat properly during pregnancy, it is not enough! Good nutrition in the man helps to ensure healthy sperm and sexual activity. A poor nutritional status in the woman can cause problems of fertility, as birthrate studies during famines have shown. (Wynn 1986, Antonov 1974, Smith 1947) The woman will need to have her body packed with all the nutrients the embryo will require to develop into a healthy fetus. Ideally she should be neither very overweight, nor underweight, since both can have adverse effects on pregnancy outcome. (Laurence 1980, Mortimer 1975, Cannon 1983, Ebrahim 1979, Rush 1980)

The importance of food during pregnancy
Women on good diets have better pregnancy outcomes than those on poor diets. (Montagu 1961, Doyle, 1990) Women who have acted upon the dietary advice they have been given also have better pregnancy outcomes than those who fail to modify their diets. (Reusens 1979) Ensuring better maternal nutrition can lower infant mortality rates(Laurence 1980). The size, and maybe function, of the child's brain is dependent on good nutrition. (Mortimer 1975)

Weight gain in pregnancy
In this situation, small is NOT beautiful! Research has shown that the old idea that a woman should not put on much weight was wrong. In a London study,

mothers in Hampstead who had higher calorie intakes than mothers in Hackney, had babies who were in some cases 2lb heavier. (Cannon 1983) Dr Ebrahim, Institute of Child Health, London, found that mothers who gained more than 30lb had the best birth outcomes. (Ebrahim 1979) Other research which has given food supplements to women has found that those who took them had bigger babies. (Rush 1980) Women who are underweight at conception, and who gain less than 11kg, or 24lb, during pregnancy, often have babies who are small-for-dates or growth retarded.

Clearly, if more is eaten without an increase in exercise a person's weight will rise. It is important not just to eat more but also to eat the right kind of foods. Besides taking in extra calories for growth and energy the mother also needs extra vitamins, minerals, essential fatty acids and amino acids. Moreover, if the correct foods are eaten, there will be less of a problem losing the weight after birth, while breast feeding, with no need for a special slimming programme.

A healthy diet

There are many misconceptions about a healthy diet. In reviewing the importance of nutrition to preconception, FORESIGHT originally drew from the work of three pioneers of nutritional research, Dr Weston Price, Sir Robert McCarrison and Dr Francis Pottenger and also that of Roger Williams, Adelle Davis, Isobel Jennings, Bert Vallee, Eric Underwood, Lucille Hurley, Donald Caldwell and Donald Oberleas.

It is really quite simple to eat properly, as any wholefood cookery book shows. The FORESIGHT Wholefood Cookbook gives good basic guidance on diet and an excellent selection of recipes, based on fresh meat and fish, fresh fruit and vegetables, fresh nuts and wholegrains. (Jervis 1984)

A good diet comprises carbohydrates, fats, proteins and clean water. Within these groups are found the various vitamins and minerals that are essential for well being. There has been so much research done on the various components that we are restricting the information in this chapter considerably, though the papers mentioned give further guidance.

Carbohydrates

should be unrefined, "with nothing added and nothing taken away!" They include starches, sugars and fibres. They provide energy. Contrary to popular belief, they are not fattening if they are eaten in the form of complex carbohydrates.

Sources: Complex carbohydrates, including whole grains (wholemeal flour, millet, wholemeal bread, oatmeal, buckwheat, brown rice, maize meal), fresh vegetables and fresh fruit.

Bad sources: Simple carbohydrates, including sugars, white flour, white bread, white pasta, sweets. These are all poor in fibre, vitamins and minerals.

Proteins

are sometimes called 'building blocks', as they are used to build or repair enzymes, muscles, organs, tissues and hair. Proteins are made of amino acids which are broken down in the body to form other amino acids. The potential of amino acids in health is only just beginning to be understood. Two amino acids, spermadine and aspermine, play a major role in the synthesis of semen (Erdmann 1987). Their levels have been found to be low in men who have low sperm counts. Fortunately, with the right foods and supplements, it is possible to raise levels and help improve sperm count. Many other factors are involved in the production of healthy sperm.

Amino acids are especially important in digestion as they form the enzymes necessary for the digestive processes. Thus if they are in short supply digestion may be effected and this may result in shortages of other nutrients in the body. Such shortages can interfere with various processes, including fertility and pregnancy. (Erdmann 1987) Animal products and fish contain all the amino acids. However to get the full range from vegetable sources it is advisable to combine nuts with pulses, nuts with seeds or pulses with seeds. Combining is an excellent way to improve the quality of protein eaten. (Moore Lappe 1975, Jervis 1984)

Sources: Fresh meat, poultry, offal, fish, milk, eggs, cheese, nuts, pulses and seeds (including whole grains).

Poor sources: Bought pies, TV meals, sausages and hamburgers, salamis, pates and other processed meats, also twice-cooked meat, as this is not fresh.

Fats

provide energy and build the cell walls. Although animal fats are sometimes linked with illnesses such as atherosclerosis and arteriosclerosis, heart disease and some cancers, both animal and vegetable fats are necessary as part of a healthy diet.

Eaten in the correct proportion and as part of a wholefood diet, there is no need to eliminate animal fats, such as butter, unless there is a specific medical reason. Polyunsaturated fats occur in vegetables, nuts, unheated vegetable oils and fish oils, all of which should be included in the diet. Monounsaturates, such as Olive oil are more beneficial in combatting Cholesterol levels. It is not generally advisable to eat margarines high in polunsaturates and often highly processed. (For those who do need alternatives to butter and cream. Jervis's book is a useful source. (Jervis 1984)

Vitamins and Minerals
are vital components of the diet and in order to express their importance they have been given whole sections of their own.

Water
Clean water is essential for health. Unfortunately there is ample evidence to show that most people do not have access to clean water. Much does not measure up to European Union standards, often having high levels of nitrates, chemicals, lead and other toxins. (Smyth 1988) Water companies have been exposed as Britain's biggest polluters. (Ryan 1994) Nitrates are known "to alter and stabilise the chemical structure of haemoglobin, so that it is unable to bind and release oxygen." They are suspected of causing stomach cancers. (Pfeiffer 1978) Heavy metals which may be found in water include lead, sometimes from old lead piping, and sometimes from water which has run off polluted land. Aluminium is even added to water as a flocculent in some areas. Mercury may come from industrial processes. (See Toxic metals)

Among the most worrying chemicals polluting water are what have been called "Oestrogen mimics". These are man-made chemicals that do not biodegrade but persist in the environment for a relatively long time. In an excellent series of reviews Max Fox.has outlined the issues. (Fox 1994a, 1994b, 1994c) The list of chemicals which mimic oestrogens is long, including (not exclusively): "pesticides eg as organochlorides – DDT + DDE, Kelthane, Heptachlor, Kepane, Methoxychlor, and the industrial chemicals eg PCBs and Bispenol A. Also EE – Oestrogen Ethyldial, herbicides, APE's – Industrial Detergents that degrade to environmentally persistent oestrogenic compounds and PCB's – which are already known to have oestrogenic properties. A completely new group of oestrogenic compounds have been found – NONYLPHENOLS". (Fox 1994a) Nonylphenol has been used widely in industry for over 40 years and is now widespread in British waters. In concentrations of only 50 micrograms it has been shown to be oestrogenic. In one unpublished study by a water authority, fish in the River Lee, England, were found to be hermaphroditic (Fox 1994a) and diseased. (Nuttall 1994d) The Royal Free Hospital whose patients include those from the river Lee area has found falling sperm quality. (Fox 1994a)

It is well known that exposure to synthetic oestrogen can cause malformations, as the DES tragedy highlighted. Fox explains the dangers for the male. After the female genital tract structure has disappeared in the male fetus

"the testes, located in the abdomen, descend into the scrotum. Sertoli cells in the testes act as a sort of nursery cell supporting

159

the cells that will produce sperm. The Sertoli cell regulates, when the testes descend, masculinisation of the reproductive tract and development of the urethra. Within the developing testes it regulates cell division – hence a possible link with testicular cancer. Excessive exposure to oestrogen, by suppressing other hormones, could reduce multiplication of Sertoli cells during foetal development."

(Fox 1994)

FORESIGHT recommends the use of a water filter. The Dalton Ceramic Filter with Supercarb cartridge will filter out the oestrogens and other pollutants. (See Appendix one) The Waymaster Crystal jug filter is recommended for kitchen use.

Pesticides

The dangers of chlorinated pesticides (organochlorides) were highlighted by Rachel Carsen in *Silent Spring* and many have now been banned though public analysts still find traces of them in foods. The most widely known is DDT, but the now banned kepone (chlordecone) and DBCP are the two best established occupational causes of male reproductive disorder. Kepone is very persistent and disposal is difficult. Severe effects of poisoning included olisgopermia. (Straub 1983) DBCP (Dibromochloropropane) caused azoospermia. (Whorton 1977)

The bans on organochlorides have lead to an increasing use of organophosphorus pesticides (organophosphate). The insecticide properties of these chemicals were discovered in 1937, although the substances on which they are based had originally been developed as potential nerve gas. Since the 1960s, formulae less toxic to man have been developed for use in pest control. But "less toxic" does not mean "not toxic", for these chemicals are increasingly being shown to have serious effects on health. This is not surprising since they work by inactivating various enzyme systems in the organisms which ingest them.(Socialist Countryside Group 1987) However, they cannot discriminate between organisms, so man is affected by them as well as the insects at which their poisonous effects are directed.

The main enzymes affected are:

1 Cholinesterase, which is responsible for hydrolysing acetylcholine from choline. Cholinesterase is found in high concentrations in the spinal cord of fetal lambs and humans during the development of the spinal cord. It only increases in the brain-stem and brain shortly before birth. (Gray's Anatomy 1954)

2 Liver enzymes. The synergistic effects of two organophosphates can be especially damaging, as can the situation where a drug is given which has toxic side effects for the liver.

3 Neurotoxic esterase (NTE). This enzyme is not only inhibited, but there will be changes in the structure and function of the affected nerves. (Roberts Undated)

Obviously substances which affect such a wide range of enzymes will result in a large variety of conditions. Target organs affected by organophosphate insecticides and nerve agent poisoning include the central nervous system, various glands, the iris, ciliary muscle, gut, bladder, heart, the autonomic ganglia and skeletal muscle. (Duffy 1980) In studies of animals and humans who have been intentionally or accidentally exposed, many effects have been reported, including ataxia, brain dysfunction, irreversible delayed neurotoxicity, damage to the nerve axon, increased secretion from the naso-lacrimal glands, bronchial glands, sweat glands, gastrointestinal glands, bronchoconstriction, cardiovascular problems such as hypotension, skeletal problems, restlessness, tremor, tonic/clonic convulsions, abnormal reflexes, respiratory and cardiac depression, coma, emotional lability, visual hallucinations, increased libido, excessive dreaming, peripheral weakness, lesions of the myelin sheath (suggesting a role in multiple sclerosis perhaps), memory loss, depression, schizophrenic reactions and inappropriate focusing of attention, long-term change in brain function and death. (Duffy 1979, Roberts Undated, Johnson 1975)

This list, long though it is, is not exhaustive. If one adds the reactions found in cattle which have been treated with organophosphorus warble fly dressing there is also: paralysis, incoordination, skin lesions, depressed milk yield, bloat, abdominal distress, excessive salivation, no remastication, anorexia, hypermotility of the intestines and diarrhoea, rapid breathing, muscle twitching, shivering, stilted movement, weakness, ataxia of the hind legs with tail head raised but the rest limp, periods of excitement and depression, bradycardia and urination. In some more severe cases the animal tends to fall around with paddling of the legs: inactivation of the body and limbs follows, with the head and neck being swung from side to side. The side effects may last for several days. One researcher has said that the incidence rate was one per 46,000 animals! (Andrews 1981)

However, not everyone agrees. Mark Purdey, a British farmer who successfully challenged the Government over their pesticide policy, argues that the incidence is much higher. (Purdey 1988) He has now suggested that Bovine Spongiform Encephalus (BSE) and other conditions of neurological damage are linked with pesticide use, a claim dismissed by government officials. (Woffinden 1994. Hornsby 1993) Yet there is support for his ideas from a number of medical experts. Researchers in a paper published by the Canadian Journal of Neurological Sciences in 1987 discovered "that a significant correlation exists between pesticide use and the prevalence of Parkinson's disease." (Woffinden 1994)

The Health and Safety Executive in the UK is monitoring possible links between pesticides, and Lindane in particular, and CHARGE syndrome. This was first described in 1979 and the acronym CHARGE first used in 1981.

Children with CHARGE syndrome exhibit at least four of the following features: Coloboma, Heart defect, choanal Atresia, growth Retardation, Genital hypoplasia and/or Ear anomalies or deafness or both. In a study of children with CHARGE it was found that some parents thought an organophosphate like Lindane could be the cause. The researchers found that "Many . . . were exposed to a number of toxins including Lindane between the 5th and 11th week of uterine life. This is a crucial stage of embryonic development. . . " (Blake 1993)

By 1995 all sheep dip users in Britain will have to have a certificate of competence. (MAFF 1994a) However, there is no enforcement of the proper disposal of dips to ensure that water supplies are not contaminated. The suspected teratogens, ioxnil and bromoxynil, are banned to all but farmers and their workers, albeit with use restricted to grass, leeks and onions. (MAFF 1994b)

Access to figures on residue levels are secret so the public does not know if foods contain harmful substances. However, the Association of Public Analysts in the UK, which conducts tests for the Government, found residues in one third of fresh fruit and vegetables it tested in 1983, and the level was regarded as significant in a seventh of all samples collected. (Young 1984) Other checks have been equally disturbing. (Erlichman 1986) In 1993 the Ministry of Agriculture, Fisheries and Food admitted that about 10 percent of UK lettuces contained the banned chemicals cholothalonil and vinclozolin. (Anon 1993)

The only sure way patients can reduce their pesticide exposure in food is to eat organically grown and reared produce. However, they must also be aware of the amount of pesticides used in other products, such as clothing and furniture. Soft furnishing materials, mattresses and bedding may be treated with moth-proofing and flame retardants. Fly sprays are a major source in the home. Flea collars on pets are impregnated with pesticides. Fungicides are used in decorating products. In the garden, wood treatments and greenhouse/plant sprays are also sources. On holiday, hotel rooms may be contaminated by mosquito repellant.

R adiation

Ionising radiation

The dangers of ionising radiation are well known, though the reasons are not always fully understood. Ionising rays are so powerful that they shatter atoms they touch, causing them to lose electrons, thereby developing an electric charge. The resulting charged particles, or ions, can penetrate the body without a person knowing, breaking up atoms and molecules to form free radicals and oxidising agents. These two chemical groups may be quite damaging in themselves, as they break up proteins, destroy chromosomes and change other chemicals. This may result in the death of cells, immediately or earlier than the usual lifespan, changes in the growth and divison of the cell such that there may be no growth or uncontrolled growth (Cancer), or prominent changes in the way the cell works.

Man has always been exposed to some ionising radiation. However, Dr Rosalie Bertell has pointed out that the "natural" levels have increased from an exposure of 60 millirems a year in 1940 to 100 in the 1950s, to 200 in the 1980s – mainly due to weapons testing. (Bertell 1986) Not all scientists agree with her figures, but no-one disputes that more of us are exposed to more radiation than ever before, not least because of an increase in the use of X-rays and nuclear medicine. There is also a large amount of low level radiation in many industries that may have seemed innocuous. Indeed, in the UK, some 6,000 sites are approved as being able to handle radioactive materials, including schools and factories. Sometimes workers are not told they are handling radioactive materials. In some areas materials are dumped without proper authority or protection for nearby residents. (Dispatches 1988)

Sometimes clinical judgement will dictate that any risks are outweighed by the benefits, as in the case of some X-rays. But no level of radiation has been proved safe, and it is likely that any level is potentially harmful. A quick look, for example, through The Bulletin of the Atomic Scientists reveals a number of studies which relate radiation dosages to malformations such as Down's syndrome, Patau's syndrome, Edward's syndrome, severe mental retardation, perinatal loss and neurological damage, to mention but a few.

(Anon 1992) Dr Bertell worries that scientists only ask about the risks of cancer from radiation when there may be other, more serious side effects. She is especially concerned about the genetic pool: "Children are now being born weakened by radioactivity, prone to enzyme disorders, allergies and asthma directly caused by cell mutations." She talks of a weakened new generation less able to cope with an ever increasing dose of radiation in the environment. "By the fifth generation of children born into the post-nuclear age the damage to the entire gene pool will be very clear indeed." She denounces the international level that power stations work to. . . "maximum 500 millirems a year to the public or plant workers. . . equivalent to 100 chest X-rays". (Bertell 1986) Other researchers have also indicated that even increases in background radioactivity, within natural levels, may have damaging effects on the fetus and may be a reason for higher malformation rates. (Ferreira 1969)

X-rays are known to create a high risk of childhood leukemia.(Bithell 1975) Animal research has confirmed this, in both males and females. When the mature eggs of female mice were irradiated the offspring had a high incidence of cancer. (Nomura 1982) Where dominant mutations have been produced in male germ cells by X-rays, low birth weight in subsequent offspring results. (Kirk 1984)

Non-ionising radiation

Non-ionising rays, including ultra violet, infra red, lasers, microwaves, radar, radio frequency waves, and extra low frequency waves are produced naturally by the sun and also created in the home, in industry and in military use. Although not powerful enough to create ions, no-one should be fooled about their safety. The chief of research of non-ionising radiation at the National Institute of Environmental Health Sciences, North Carolina, Donald McCree has said:

> "In animal experiments, (the Russians) have found that this radiation causes changes in almost every system: behaviour, blood chemistry, the endocrine functions, reproductive organs, and the immune system. In studies of human workers exposed to microwave equipment for many years, they have reported abnormally slow heart beats, chest pains, and birth defects. And they've found a lot of more subjective effects, things like insomnia, irritability, headaches, and loss of memory."
>
> (McCree Undated)

Visual Display Units – VDUs

VDUs are widely used in the workplace and home. There is considerable debate over their safety, especially for the pregnant woman but few conclusions can be drawn. Studies have produced mixed results, though one reason may be that the testing is not always done on machines as they are used – perhaps neglected, unserviced and without proper safety precautions. They may release low levels of radiation, including X-rays, microwaves, ultra violet and infra red light. (Bonnell 1984) Although some authorities argue that these levels are too low to cause harm, Tony Webb, a noted expert on the subject, disagrees:

> "There is no safe level of radiation. In addition, there is no conclusive evidence that these low levels do not cause damage."
> (Webb 1984)

Worries about birth defects and VDUs arose from reports of an apparently high number of birth defects among a group of VDU operators in Canada in 1980. Other studies have revealed clusters, including one among staff at the Department of Employment in Cheshire, UK, where in 55 pregnancies in VDU users, 14.5 per cent ended with a miscarriage, 6.7 per cent in stillbirth and 22 per cent in some kind of malformation. For women not using VDUs the figures were 5.3 per cent, less than 1 per cent and 11 per cent respectively. (Webb 1984) However, there were reservations about the statistics. It may be that VDU operators suffer high levels of stress, especially if they work for long uninterrupted periods. Stress is known to be a risk factor in pregnancy. In 1988 a large-scale epidemiological study on computer users reported on 1,583 pregnant women.

> "The results showed that female workers using computers more than twenty hours per week had twice the miscarriage rate of female workers who did similar work but did not use the computers. While the number of birth defects in the entire group was too small for accurate statistical analysis, the team reported that women using terminals more than twenty hours a week have a 40 per cent increased incidence of miscarriage compared with non users."
> (Anon 1985)

Besides the risk of miscarriage, one researcher has also reported a number of other conditions associated with VDUs, including birth defects in the children of operators, disturbances in menstrual cycle, and general symptoms associated with chronic stress – headache, nausea, sleeplessness and fatigue. (DeMatteo 1985) In some countries, notably Scandinavia and the USA, employers are seeking ways of limiting their employees' exposure to VDU radiation. (Goldhaber 1988) This can be done by regular rest periods, protective equipment to reduce the rays, and shielding of the operator with special clothing. The latter, however, does not protect organs such as the thyroid. Robert Becker, the leading authority on the effects of electromedicine, suggests that one should place the computer proper, its monitor and peripherals at least 30 inches from the keyboard and desist from using computers during pregnancy. (Becker 1990)

It would seem sensible if these precautions were standard procedure, since with what is known about low level radiation, it is unlikely that there will be conclusive proof that VDUs are not potentially harmful. Preconception couples need to be aware of the risks.

Microwaves

Microwaves can penetrate deeply into the body, causing its temperature to rise. High intensity microwaves can lead to permanent damage. For example, the heat generated can cause the cell lining of the testicles to degenerate, thereby damaging them. (Anon 1980a) It is also suspected of causing breast cancer, especially where a microwave oven is placed at breast height. (Schauss 1986) The problem arises because the breast and the eyes have a poor blood supply so the heat is not dissipated. Microwaves may also cause genetic damage: One study has shown that more Down's syndrome children were fathered by men exposed to microwaves than by fathers not so exposed. (Stellman 1979)

Electromagnetic fields

> ". . . All abnormal, man-made electromagnetic fields, regardless of their frequencies, produce the same biological effects."   (Becker 1990)

Having made this statement Becker goes on to explain that these effects, deviations from normal functions and "actually or potentially harmful", include "effects on growing cells. . . developmental abnormalities in embryos. . . alterations in neurochemicals, resulting in behavioural abnormalities such as suicide, alterations in biological cycles, stress responses in exposed animals that, if prolonged, lead to declines in immune-system efficiency. . . "

The adverse effects of electromagnetic fields have been known for many years, though officials have sometimes been dismissive of any dangers. (Wright 1988) Russia limited the time a farm worker can spend near high-voltage power lines to three hours, while the USA will not allow houses to be built near them. (Anon 1988) One group of researchers found an increase in all birth defects for conceptions that occurred during the time the father worked on high-voltage systems. (Nordstrom 1981) Men working in high-voltage switching yards were found to father more congenitally malformed children than would be expected. (Nordstrom 1983) A number of animal studies have reported health problems, including fetal abnormalities. (Becker 1990) Dr Nancy Wertheimer and her colleagues suggested an association between the use of electric blankets and infertility and birth defects. They hypothesised that strong electromagnetic fields may be generated by electric blankets under certain circumstances. The seasonal variation of rates of births and birth defects may agree with the time periods of peak electric blanket use. (Wertheimer 1984)

(Of course, they may also peak with many other factors such as reduced sunlight or different food availability.) Dr Wertheimer has also undertaken a study showing that women living in homes in which electric heating cables have been installed in the ceilings have higher rates of miscarriage. (Becker 1990)

Tests during Pregnancy

Doctors have a number of tests available to them to assist in monitoring pregnancy. Some of these are discussed in the section on the preconception medical check and are conducted before pregnancy. Some, including blood pressure and some blood tests, are also conducted during pregnancy. Some are only conducted during pregnancy to monitor the health of the fetus, checking mainly for congenital abnormalities and genetic disorders. The tests should be supportive of genetic counselling and not a substitute for it, though the tendency now is to offer them as routine. It is advisable to note that ALL tests need careful thought; ALL tests carry risks in themselves, so the use of them should be minimised. Once advised upon the risks of the tests it is the patient's responsibility to decide whether or not to have them.

General advice for doctors at the preconception stage

The need for tests should be considerably reduced if the FORESIGHT medical protocol is followed, incorporating the following during preconception counselling:

Minerals status ensured;

Toxic metals reduced;

All infections and infestations, especially genito-urinary, toxoplasmosis, CMV and candidiasis fully treated;

No smoking or alcohol or other drugs taken for four months before and during pregnancy;

Oral contraception abandoned six month prior to conception;

Rubella immunity check;

Allergies cleared.

The doctor may wish to explain that the preconception care programme as suggested by FORESIGHT is concerned with the prevention of defects, so if it is followed, the chances of an abnormal pregnancy are minimised.

Ideally thought should be given to testing in general before conception. It is difficult for the patient to be objective during pregnancy, especially if in the event of an unfortunate outcome, abortion has to be considered. This can be even more difficult if a choice has to be made after the result of a test such as amniocentesis, where the pregnancy will be quite advanced. It is advisable to discuss attitudes to abortion during preconception counselling. Tests should only be considered when there is an increased risk of severe genetic disorder or birth defect for which there is little or no effective treatment, such as in Down's syndrome or neural tube defects. Family history may indicate other risks, such as haemophilia. Very serious consideration should be given to the risk of miscarriage linked with many of the tests in older women, especially those over 40 years of age, carrying a much wanted baby, as the chances of another conception may be less at this age.

Operator experience is important in many of the tests – the more experienced the operator, the greater the safety and efficacy of the test.

Amniocentesis

This should not be a routine test and should be offered only where there is a high risk to the fetus. Such cases would include situations where the mother may be the carrier of a genetically linked disorder such as haemophilia or muscular dystrophy, or be at risk of a baby with a chromosomal abnormality, such as Down's syndrome. The test may also be done if her AFP level is high or if she will need a Caesarean section. The test should always be done with an ultrasound scan to ensure that the needle is in the right place to minimise the risks of piercing the fetus. Thus in considering the risks of amniocentesis one also needs to take into account the risks of ultrasound scans.

It is difficult to assess the risks of this test, though they are often quoted as about 1.5 per cent risk of miscarriage (in addition to the normal risk of miscarriage). The studies that have been done are mostly flawed in some way when one tries to assess the results statistically, as there are many factors which can cause fetal loss which cannot be taken into account when doing the research but which may raise the risk figures. However, in their excellent review of all the studies done up to 1986, Ager and Oliver say that overall, the results indicate that there is a real risk to the fetus. They report on research done in Denmark which they claim was the best study undertaken to date. In this the rate of spontaneous abortion was significantly higher than in the control group, being 1.7 per cent to 0.7 per cent. (Ager 1986)

It is sometimes claimed that the adverse effects to the woman appear to be very small, though it is hard to understand, since any risk to the fetus must affect the woman. (Turnbull 1984) These risks include fetal death, miscarriage, vaginal bleeding followed by miscarriage, and stillbirth. The risks seem to be increased if the obstetrician is not skilled. This is not surprising when one considers that the two main events which cause fetal death are needle damage and the introduction of infection. (Ager 1986) Other risks listed in the Medical

Research Council report include an increased incidence of neonatal respiratory distress in about 3 per cent of offspring and an increased number of congenital dislocations of the hip and talipes in 2.4 per cent of offspring.(Medical Research Council 1978) More recently early amniocentesis has become an alternative to chorionic villus sampling (CVS) but a trial to compare the two techniques was abandoned after it was found that the miscarriage rate was twice as high among those having amniocentesis. (Stuttaford 1994d) "In evaluating the benefits of amniocentesis it should not be forgotten that the indications are relative and the risks not insignificant." (Ritchie 1982)

Barts' or Triple (Marker) Test
This is a recent development and still the subject of much debate as it only detects about 60 per cent of Down's syndrome pregnancies, though one publication claims a 91 per cent detection rate. (Green 1993)

Maternal alpha fetoprotein – commonly called AFP
This is done 16 weeks into the pregnancy, so a doctor needs to be certain of dates if it is to be helpful. About 2 per cent of women have a raised level of alpha fetoprotein, of whom only about 1 in 20 has real problems. In others it may be a multiple pregnancy or the pregnancy may be more advanced than was thought. (Dixon 1980) There could be an error at the laboratory. Some research has suggested a failure rate of 20 per cent. In this the AFP level was not raised but subsequently a baby was born with a neural tube defect. (Harris 1981) It is also known for normal babies to have been born to mothers with high AFP levels. (Sutton 1988)

Chorionic villus biopsy
The main advantage quoted of this test is that it can be done in the first three months of pregnancy, allowing time for an early abortion. However, there are a number of risks. Immediate complications can include perforations of the amniotic sac, severe bleeding (rare), mild to moderate bleeding in under 10 per cent of cases, infection, and feto-maternal haemorrhage leading to isoimmunisation. (Loeffler 1985) There is an increased risk of miscarriage, but it is difficult to assess. (Haire 1983) 2-3 per cent is quoted, but this should not be taken as accurate. Indeed, one study assesses the risk for transcervical biopsy as much higher. London hospital experience suggests a miscarriage rate of over 10 per cent, though the figures in other studies vary between 3 and 30 per cent. From a total of 91 patients tested using the transabdominal route there was only one miscarriage. (Lilford 1985) However, there is no mention in the study of the health of the neonate, nor of subsequent development. Evidence of a link between CVS and limb reduction has been accumulating from around the world. (Firth 1994, Dispatches 1995) More

than 40 babies have been damaged in the 30,000 CVS procedures done in the UK up to 1995. The evidence suggests that the earlier the CVS is performed, the greater the risk of limb reduction, with the risk declining sharply in the 11th week of pregnancy. WHO and British guidelines say that CVS is safe from the ninth week of pregnancy, though this is disputed by experts who have looked at the accumulating data on limb reduction. One suggests that CVS should not be performed until the 12th week. (Nikolaides 1995) There is a strong correlation with ora-mandibular limb hypogenesis syndrome. (Mastroiacovo 1995) False negatives been reported. (Lilford 1991a, Lilford 1991b) Fetal exsanguination has also been reported, leading to fetal death. (Froas 1993)

Operator experience is important. One study of work on one operator on 3016 patients showed a total of 99.7 per cent good samples. However, for the first one hundred patients, in only 57 per cent was the sample achieved with a single insertion. In the next 2516 patients the rate was 96 per cent. The number of insertions is crucial, since with one insertion the loss in the first and second trimester of pregnancies planned to continue was 1.94 per cent, rising to 6.4 per cent where three insertions had taken place. (Williams 1992) The WHO suggests that an operator may need 250 practices before being ready to work unsupervised. (Dispatches 1995) Doctors at one London hospital believe that with an experienced operator, CVS is as safe as late amniocentesis, and very much safer than amniocentesis done in the first three months of pregnancy. (Stuttaford 1994d)

Fetoscopy

This test should only be done where there is a high risk to the fetus as it is a dangerous technique for the fetus. The rate of miscarriage is said by one authority to be 3 per cent, though it could be higher. (Brooks 1982) The incidence of other risks is not known but the possibility of infections being introduced by the method cannot be ruled out.

Ultrasound scanning

When one considers the many uses to which ultrasound scanning can be put it is not surprising that it is so widely performed. Indeed, there are some doctors who advocate scanning every pregnant woman as a precaution – though one must query the nature of the precaution. Is it for the doctor's protection or the fetus'? Many women are now offered more than one scan during their pregnancy though not all doctors agree with this frequency. Some obstetricians believe that seeing the fetus can help bonding between mother and baby, even before birth, though this has been happening in other ways for centuries! Certainly a scan will increase the safety of amniocentesis, as well as revealing abnormalities, growth retardation, the presence of more than one fetus and any growths in the mother which may impede delivery. However, the test is not without its risks, and is not 100 per cent successful.

Where it is being used to reveal abnormalities, it is best done around 18-20 weeks. The doctor should be aware that false positives do occur. (Atkins 1991) A success rate of 74 per cent has been reported. (Chitty 1993) Another analysis concluded that ultrasound "does not improve outcome of pregnancy in terms of increased number of live births or of reduced perinatal mortality." (Burcher 1993)

A worrying development is the use of the transvaginal probe which exposes the fetus to higher levels of ultrasound even earlier in pregnancy than the transabdominal ultrasound. (Gullen 1990) Ultrasound waves are a form of non-ionising radiation and although they are said to be safe, especially now that very weak waves are used, this has yet to be proved. The American College of Radiology has spoken out against routine use in its Commission on Ultrasound. (American College of Radiology 1981)

The US government agency, the National Center for Radiological Health of the Food and Drug Administration, published a report saying,

> "We can be reasonably certain that acute, dramatic effects are not likely. . . But studies have not been made to detect less obvious effects, and the question of subtle, long-term or cumulating effects has not been systemmatically explored, and the potential for delayed effects has been virtually ignored".
>
> (National Center for Radiological Health 1982)

The two main hazards of ultrasound are heat and cavitation. It is thought that the rises in temperature are too small to cause damage as little heat is produced in pulsed waves of ultrasound. Cavitation, in which air bubbles expand and contract in response to the sound waves, may occur in humans, producing, among other effects, the release of free radicals. (Crum 1986) Doris Haire, the President of the American Foundation for Maternal and Child Health at a symposium in 1983, quoted studies suggesting premature ovulation after ovarian ultrasound, damage to maternal blood cells, a higher incidence of leukemia in exposed children, and lower birth weight. (Haire 1983) However, the results of some of the studies are not significant and there are problems with the research methods. Another researcher has suggested that "animal studies have been reported to reveal delayed neuro-muscular development, altered emotional behaviour, EEG changes, anomalies and decreased survival." (Finkel 1979)

The Consumers Association in the UK has said, "Women who are offered a routine scan should be informed not only why it is recommended, but also that it is not an essential part of their antenatal care." (Consumers Association 1985) FORESIGHT supports this position. The data on risks is limited, but "absence of proof is not proof of absence."

X-rays (See radiation)
Before any X-ray ensure that there is absolutely no alternative and that it is essential to the well-being of the mother and the fetus.

Toxic Metals – also known as Heavy Metals

All trace elements can be toxic if consumed in sufficient quantities. However, the term "toxic metal" generally denotes "those elements not recognised as having an essential function and known to have well documented deleterious effects." (Lodge Rees, 1983b)

Man has been utilising these metals for hundreds of years, but in this century new processes, purposes and products have meant an escalation in use. The result is widespread pollution with sometimes serious effects on health. The injurious effects of lead were recognised with the introduction of lead-free petrol, though its use is still far from universal. Although the dangers of cadmium are highlighted in discussions on soil levels, there is little apparent concern over its major sources, cigarette smoking and refined flours. Dentists have been aware of the risks of mercury yet continue to use amalgam fillings. The possible toxicity of aluminium has been highlighted in respect of Alzheimer's Disease, but UK hospitals, especially those dealing with the mentally ill and geriatrics, serve large amounts of tea, a high source of aluminium. The use of deodorants and anti-perspirants grows as it becomes anti-social to smell human, and these are also often high in aluminium salts.

A further problem is the continual interaction between the elements in the body – though it is the relationship between the individual elements that is important in health. Unfortunately there are only a small number of studies which review these interactional effects as the work is difficult and expensive; Bryce-Smith and his colleagues have pursued it. (Ward, 1987) These are discussed in more detail below. There is also the problem common to government health departments and the medical industry; the assumption that something is safe until it is proved otherwise. What is needed is a major shift to assume the opposite, namely that something with toxic potential is dangerous until proved safe!

The major toxic metals which are known to influence pregnancy outcome include lead, cadmium, aluminum, mercury and copper and these are reviewed in more detail below. Other metals have been brought under suspicion as embryotoxic or teratogenic in animal tests. Arsenic has been found

175

to act as a transplacental carcinogen. (Elkington 1985) A study among workers in Sweden has implicated it in decreased birth weight and an increased rate of spontaneous abortion, but the design of the study was poor so the results are subject to debate. Depending on when it is taken into the body, it is said it can cause neural tube defects, agenesis and renal problems. (Mortensen 1986)

Aluminium

Sources: The major sources of aluminium include antacids, antiperspirants and food additives, especially an anti-caking agent found in milk substitutes. In some places aluminium flocculants are added to the water, so if a patient's hair level is high, the water from their tap should be tested as a priority. Aluminium saucepans and other cooking utensils impart some metal if they are in contact with food. Leaf vegetables, rhubarb, apple and other acid fruits are especially problematic. Pressure cookers are worse than ordinary pans. Kettles and aluminium teapots are potent sources, especially if the tea is allowed to stand for a long time. Work at the University of Wales at Cardiff suggests that the major UK food source of aluminium is tea, since the tea plant thrives on alum soils, so the soil is fed with alum. Foil-wrapped foods, such as meats, fish, poultry and pies made in foil saucers are other sources. Foil-wrapped fats and acid foods are the worst. (Pfeiffer 1978, Millstone 1988)

Effects on health: Aluminium is easily absorbed, accumulating in the arteries. A study has shown that people living in areas with a high level of aluminium in the drinking water face a 50 per cent greater risk of developing Alzeimher's Disease. It is known that aluminium can destroy vitamins as it readily combines with other substances. It weakens the lining of the gut. It inhibits fluorine and phosphorus metabolism, resulting in mineral loss from the bones over a long period. Excessive amounts can lead to constipation, colic, excessive perspiration, loss of appetite, nausea, skin problems and fatigue. Adverse effects associated with the body's attempts to clear itself, in which aluminium salts are found in small quantities in the blood, include paralysis and areas of numbness, with fatty degeneration of the liver and kidney, as well as symptoms of gastrointestinal inflammation. Thus it seriously compromises nutritional status. It has been linked with kidney problems in babies, with researchers concluding that formula feeds should be aluminium-free for neonates and infants with reduced kidney function. It has been associated with behavioural problems and autism. Mice fed large doses had no symptoms, but the next three generations of offspring had growth defects. (Cowdry 1989, Nutrition Search Inc 1975, Freundlich 1985, Lodge Rees 1979, Ward 1992)

FORESIGHT recommends that the Hair Mineral analysis level should not exceed 2 parts per million.

Cadmium

Sources: The main sources of cadmium are cigarette smoking and processed foods, since in the refining of flour the zinc in the germ and bran layers is removed, leaving a high cadmium to zinc ratio. It is also found in water, especially where impure zinc has been used in galvanising of pipes and mains through which soft water flows. It is widely used in manufacturing industries, including those concerned with paint, batteries, television sets and fertilisers. It is found in shellfish from polluted waters and galvanised containers and coal-burning. It is a common pollutant which is highly dangerous as it accumulates in the kidneys and liver slowly, unless nutritional measures are taken to remove it or reduce absorption. It particularly builds up in people who are deficient of Vitamins C, D, B6, zinc, manganese, copper, selenium and/or calcium. (Pfeiffer 1978, McKie 1983, Colgan 1982, Pfeiffer 1975)

Effects on health : Cadmium is known to be embryotoxic in animals. Elizabeth Lodge Rees has reported cleft palate and/or lip, other facial malformations and limb defects in a number of species, testicular and ovarian necrosis, and renal disorders. Pregnant animals have developed toxemia, an observation which has lead her to wonder if "one might suspect that toxemia in humans may be due to excess cadmium and/or a lack of nutrients that counteract the effect of cadmium". She also mentioned that in humans it is associated with proteinuria as well as low birth weight and small head circumference. Cadmium accumulates in the placenta, causing placental necrosis if large amounts are absorbed. (Lodge Rees 1983b) It also crosses the placenta. It has been found to impair reproduction in mice. (Bryce Smith 1981, Schroeder 1971)

The importance of zinc in counteracting the effects of cadmium has been demonstrated in animal research on the effects of cadmium on the testes. Pretreatment with zinc can abolish some of the adverse effects, though it does not reverse others. When cadmium is injected subcutaneously into female rats it produces marked changes in the ovaries, the adverse effects initially increasing over time, though the ovaries do return to normal eventually. (Samarawickrama 1983)

FORESIGHT recommends that the hair mineral analysis level should not exceed 0.15 parts per million.

Copper

(an essential mineral, but over-high levels can be harmful)

Sources: The contraceptive pill and copper coil can both cause copper levels in the body to rise. (Grant 1985) In soft water areas, or where the water has been heated through an Ascot heater, the water may contain high levels of copper. The kettle or pan should always be filled from the cold tap. If the patient has been using a water filter for two weeks and sees the white contents of the filter change to blueish green there is likely to be a significantly high level of copper and the water should be checked. Filtering should continue with the filter cartridge being changed regularly. Copper kettles, pans and jewelry are also sources. There may be external contamination of hair samples by Henna dyes and rinses, and from swimming-pool water where the pool has been treated with a copper-containing algicide. For an accurate hair reading the patient should cease the contamination for six weeks before having a further hair mineral analysis.

Effects on Health: Excessive levels of copper may be embryotoxic or teratogenic. They are known to produce behavioural symptoms, such as uncontrollable rages and are linked with toxemia. Copper levels rise naturally during pregnancy, so if a woman conceives with a raised level she is at risk of overloading her body. This could lead to postpartum depression. High copper levels have been linked to premature birth in a number of animal studies. Raised levels are associated with low levels of manganese and zinc, deficiencies of which are known to cause birth defects. (See Minerals) (Elkington 1985, Pfeiffer 1978, Norwood 1980, Vallee 1965)

FORESIGHT recommends a hair reading of no more than 15–20 ppm to start a pregnancy.

Lead

Lead has been known to be toxic to animals and humans for centuries and its use is now so great that it is impossible to escape ingesting or inhaling it.

Sources: It comes mainly from the atmosphere, polluted by exhaust fumes from lead in petrol It is found in foods, especially those grown in soil polluted by lead from petrol, and from unlined cans. (Ward 1987, Colgan 1982) Water which has coursed though old lead piping, or through lead-glazed earthenware mains, or through modern copper piping where the joins of the pipes have been formed with lead-containing alloys, is also a major source for many people. Indeed, where a high lead level is noted in a hair mineral test, the water should be checked as a first line of enquiry. Cigarette smoking can increase lead uptake by 25 per cent, partly because of the way in which it interacts with other substances, and also from the lead arsenate used as an insecticide in the production of tobacco. Occupational exposure can be a hazard, as lead is used in a number of industries. (Davis 1981, Pfeiffer 1978, Clausen 1977, El-Dakhakny 1972)

Animal research suggests that nutritional status may be a factor in lead absorption. Diets low in calcium, iron, zinc and manganese may actually enhance lead uptake. However, one study also suggests that cow's milk may increase absorption, since although it is high in calcium, it is low in other trace minerals such as iron. (Kostial, 1979) The fact that lead can be removed from the body by nutrients further supports the idea that nutritional status in important.

Safety levels: There is no agreement on safety levels of lead in the body. Some researchers say that no level can be assumed to be safe, while the Government sets limits for industry and the environment which are lowered from time to time as more is revealed about its toxicity. (Bryce Smith 1979) One problem in deciding toxicity levels is that there are no agreed ways to measure levels. Blood levels are not reliable as the lead is passed quickly into other tissues, especially bones. Hair analysis, now accepted as a reliable guide, is available through FORESIGHT, using laboratories at the University of Surrey. (No direct contact may be made to the University)
FORESIGHT recommends that the hair reading should be no more than 1 part per million.

Effects of lead toxicity on health: It is now accepted that levels of lead in the body which do not manifest symptoms of "classical lead poisoning" may have subtle effects on the body. Chronic "low" lead exposure is implicated as a significant causative or contributory factor in a wide range of conditions, including cardiovascular disease, renal and metabolic disease, immune dysfunction, and a multiplicity of vague symptoms, such as lethargy, depression, muscle aches and pains, frequent infections, cancer, developmental abnormalities and learning, behavioural and central nervous system dysfunction. Lead interferes with the normal functioning of many trace elements, especially by inhibiting zinc dependent enzymes, making its effects widespread. Other enzyme systems are also vulnerable. High childhood blood levels and smaller stature have been shown to be highly correlated.

Lead can affect both male and female reproductive abilities. Men exposed to high levels in their work have been found to be at risk of low sperm count, with more sperm likely to be misshapen and less mobile. High rates of infertility, miscarriage, stillbirth, congenital abnormalities including microcephaly, convulsions, early deaths and chromosomal alterations have been reported. In women, its capacity for inducing abortions has long been known – it was used for this purpose about the turn of the century with, sometimes, blindness and brain damage in surviving babies as unwanted results. It was also this property that ensured women were not employed to work with lead.

One reason it may be abortifacient lies in its tendency to accumulate in the placenta. In 1977, a study of placental lead levels showed that there were greater amounts in the placentas of malformed stillbirths and neonatal deaths

179

compared with normal babies surviving longer than a week. In the same year, two other researchers reported higher levels of lead (and cadmium) in stillbirths, using rib and pre-ossified cartilage for the analyses. They concluded: "Although some levels were low, others were so high as to raise the suspicion that they were aetiologically connected with the death of the fetus." Needleman and his colleagues found that the relationship between lead exposure in utero and congenital abnormalities to be associated "in a dose-related fashion with an increased risk for minor abnormalities." (Needleman 1984)

Prenatal exposure can result in lead intoxication in the new-born. In a study which measured the level of lead in umbilical cord blood at birth, subsequent mental developmental testing at the ages of 6 months and 12 months showed that the higher the level of lead the lower the test scores. At neither age were scores related to current blood levels. The researchers concluded: "Prenatal exposure to lead levels relatively common among urban populations appear to be associated with less favourable development through the first year of life." (Bellinger 1986) Another longitudinal study by the same researcher, which concerned lead exposure and early cognitive development, concluded, "It appears that the fetus may be adversely affected at blood lead concentrations well below 25 ug/dl, the level currently defined by the Center for Disease Control as the highest acceptable level for young children." (Bellinger 1987)

Research by Doctors McConnell and Berry suggest why this should happen. They found that in rats lead tends to derange the development of the brain in a special way, interrupting the process of forming neural connections. Other studies have shown that other parts of the brain closely involved with learning processes are also susceptible to damage by lead. Animal research with monkeys has confirmed that learning abilities are affected. In one study, monkeys in their first year of life showed no physical signs of toxicity, but all the lead-treated ones showed performance deficits on reversal learning tasks. The researchers report that the effects are not the result of delayed maturation:

> ". . . Data currently being collected in this laboratory indicate that the deficit can be observed at least three years beyond the final dosing. It therefore appears likely that this deficit represents a relatively permanent characteristic of the chronically lead poisoned monkey." (Bushell 1977)

The most widely quoted study on the effects of lead on children is that done by Needleman and his colleagues. They showed that at levels below those which were considered to produce symptoms of toxicity, the performance of children in the classroom was adversely affected. A wide range of behaviours was examined, including distractibility, persistence, dependence, organisational ability, hyperactivity, impulsiveness, frustration, day dreaming, ability to follow, and overall functioning, and it was found that the higher the lead level, the poorer the performance in every measure. Other studies have also indicated the negative effects of lead on learning abilities and classroom behaviour. In a follow-up study, Needleman and his colleagues checked 132 students over an 11 year period, concluding that the harmful effects of lead persist beyond childhood and the mental impairment from lead poisoning may be permanent. Decreased hand-eye co-ordination and shortened reaction times, as well as physical effects were seen in 45 adolescents and young adults with hair levels considered to be normal, with problems starting at levels as low as 10 ppm. Most laboratories class up to 15 ppm as "normal".

A number of other studies have also suggested a link between hyperactivity and raised lead levels. In one, 13 children with no apparent cause for their hyperactivity were examined. Their behaviour improved when their lead levels were reduced using lead-chelating medication. A Danish study linked high levels with minimal cerebral dysfunction (MCD) – learning disabilities are often linked with hyperactivitiy or MCD.

(Davis 1981, Blamer 1980, Lacranjan 1975, Elkington 1985, Needleman 1984, Ward 1987, Wibberley 1977, Singh 1978, Bellinger 1986, Bryce Smith 1979, Needleman 1979, Pihl 1977, Garnys 1979, Thatcher 1982, Yale 1985, Moore 1975, Gittelman 1983, Lin-Fu 1973, David 1976, Hansen 1980, Needleman 1990, Schwartz 1986)

Mercury

Sources: The main sources of mercury are pesticide and fungicides, fish, industrial process and dental fillings. The larger the fish, the greater the concentration, with tuna fish being the most likely source in the UK. Freshwater fish can also be contaminated if the river has been polluted by factory effluent, or water run off fields which have been subjected to mercury-containing agrochemicals. It is found in slimicides used in paper manufacturing to stop the growth of slime moulds.

The major controversy around the dangers of mercury concerns mercury-containing amalgams used in dentistry. (Ziff 1985, Kupsinel 1984) Dentists have been aware of mercury poisoning for many years – the American Society of Dental Surgeons was opposed to them 150 years ago! Sweden now bans mercury in dental work on pregnant women as a prelude to a total ban.

It appears that some large marine mammals ingest high levels of selenium. This detoxifies mercury, especially if taken with Vitamin E.

Effects on health: There are three basic forms of mercury, elemental, non-organic and organic. The elemental and non-organic forms tend to be slowly absorbed and readily excreted, unlike the organic form which is easily absorbed and slow to be eliminated. Thus the main dangers lie in the organic, especially methyl mercury, although there are some conditions linked to elemental mercury. These include psychological disturbances, oral cavity disorders, gastro-intestinal, cardiovascular, neurologic, respiratory, immunological and endocrine effects. In severe cases there are hallucinations and manic-depression, Organic mercury exposure is linked with psychological symptoms which develop into paralysis, vision, speech and hearing problems, loss of memory, lack of coordination, renal damage and general central nervous system dysfunctions. Eventually coma and death can occur.

Metallic mercury vapour has been reported to affect men exposed to it in a serious way. In one study of nine men, exposed after an accident, all complained of loss of libido, lasting in some cases up to eight years. One reported temporary impotence for eighteen months.

The damage mercury can cause to the fetus was highlighted in the Japanese tragedy of Minamata, in which 23 children were born with cerebral palsy-like symptoms, varying from mild spasticity to severe mental retardation, blindness, chronic seizures, and death. Their mothers, free from symptoms themselves, had been exposed to mercury while pregnant. Mercury is readily passed through the placenta and fetal blood often contains concentrations 20 per cent greater than the maternal blood. Fetal brain tissue concentrations may be four times higher than the mother's brain tissues. Adults and older children were also affected with a total of 46 dying.

Animal work by Dr Joan Spyker suggests that the adverse effects may be long-term. Mice exposed in utero did not appear outwardly different from controls until they were about 18 months old (middle-aged). The experimental mice then contracted severe infections, implying an immune system impaired prenatally. They lost all pretence of normality, ageing quickly and prematurely. Only extensive investigation, magnifying the brain tissues 48,000 times, showed slight damage to the individual cells – yet this slight damage was responsible for their problems. Dr Spyker has pointed out that the Minamata victims are deteriorating just as the animal model predicted. (Elkington 1985, Kupsinel 1984, Norwood 1980)

Multi Element Studies

As far back as 1969 it was reported that "Cadmium teratogenicity is dramatically augmented by lead when they are administered concurrently." (Thatcher 1982) Lead and cadmium often occur together. Their concentrations in hair and blood show strong positive correlations and their overt symptoms of toxicity are not unalike. These similarities have led some researchers to the view that "it is possible that some of the deleterious effects attributed to lead in correlational studies may instead be due to cadmium." They conducted a study on hair cadmium and lead levels in relation to cognitive functioning in children, in which the results showed that hair cadmium and lead levels were significantly correlated with intelligence tests and school achievement, but not with motor impairment scores. Statistical analysis suggested that "cadmium has a stronger effect on verbal IQ than does lead and that lead has a stronger effect on performance IQ than does cadmium." (Thatcher 1982)

Professor Bryce-Smith and his colleagues, aware of the inadequacies of single element studies, reviewed the levels of four elements, lead, cadmium, zinc and calcium, in stillbirths' bones and cartilage. They found that cadmium concentrates in the stillbirths were ten times greater than the levels normally found in human bones. Lead levels were also raised. Low calcium and zinc were sometimes associated with these marked elevations. (Bryce -Smith 1977)

Research has shown that lead and cadmium can also cause problems for the neonate. A much larger study by Bryce-Smith and his colleagues studied 36 elements. In 1981, Professor Bryce-Smith reported that for all the elements being studied, the levels of fetal and maternal blood were about the same for most elements. Only in lead levels was there a difference, with the fetal level about 95% of the maternal. He explained this thus:

> "This means that the placenta passes all elements, both nutrients and toxins, to the fetus from the maternal circulation with little or no selectivity or filtering effect. We can see no evidence for a significant barrier to protect the fetus from inorganic toxins such as mercury, arsenic, and antimony; and there is only a slight, but significant (p=0.01) barrier in the case of lead for normal births only."   (Bryce-Smith 1979)

Having begun by analysing nine tissues, including maternal and fetal (umbilical) cord whole blood and serum, amniotic fluid, placenta, and scalp hair from the mother and neonate, later on they decided that the placental element levels showed the clearest correlations with indices of fetal development for supposedly "normal" births. Thus it was with this tissue that they continued the investigation.

In the first written report on the final 37 elements studied, the researchers observed highly significant negative relationships between placental cadmium and lead levels, and birth weight, head circumference and placental weight. The smaller the birth weight, head circumference and placental weight was, the higher the level of cadmium and lead. There was a statistically significant positive correlation between placental cadmium and lead levels where birth weights were less than 3,000 g. For higher birth weights, the correlation, though still positive, was not significant. Placental zinc showed significant positive relationships with birth weights up to 3,000 g and head circumference of less than 34 cm, ie the lower the level of zinc, the lower the birth weight and the smaller the head circumference. With respect to other elements, there was "a weak positive correlation between placental iron and head circumference, and stronger but negative correlations for chlorine, vanadium, and lanthanum." However, placental levels of iron did not correlate with birth weight, nor were the iron levels or birth weights significantly raised in those mothers receiving iron supplements. Indeed, the results in iron and zinc lead the researchers to suggest that more emphasis should be paid to zinc supplementation than to iron. The final point made in the paper states that, "In cases of cadmium, lead, and zinc, biological, neurobehavioural, and biosocial studies in which the levels of all three elements are measured may prove more informative than those involving single elements." (Ward 1987)

Much the same conclusion was reached by the researchers who conducted further investigation into lead, cadmium, and cognitive functioning. Looking at the protective effects of zinc and calcium against toxic metals, they found that higher zinc levels seemed to protect against the effects of cadmium, while calcium did the same against lead. They concluded: "The results suggest that the effects of heavy metal pollutants on cognitive function cannot be adequately assessed without concurrently evaluating the status of essential nutrients with which these toxins are known to interact metabolically." (Lester 1986)

The most recent FORESIGHT research, conducted by the University of Surrey, is discussed in detail in the Minerals section.

Detoxifying the Body

The preferred method of detoxification must be nutritional since it does not have the same potential for side effects as drugs. EDTA can be used in acute poisoning but it is not recommended. It binds to the elements so they are removed from the body along with the EDTA, but it also removes the essential minerals.

The following is a guide to the nutrients and foods that are helpful in removing toxic metals.

Vitamin C and zinc supplements were used successfully in reducing blood lead levels of psychiatric outpatients in one study. The treatment was also found to reduce blood copper levels. Subjects included some hyperactive children. (Lester 1986) Vitamin C has also been shown to lower cadmium levels in birds. (Sohler 1977)

Calcium helps prevent absorption, as well as removing lead from the tissues. Vitamin D is necessary for calcium metabolism and to help displace lead from the bones. Vitamin B1, taken with a B-complex, provides protection against lead damage. Lecithin can also help in protection, while Vitamin A helps to activate the enzymes needed for detoxification. Trace elements, in addition to zinc, which are protective include chromium and manganese. Tablets are often used but they need to be combined with manganese to preserve its levels. In the diet, peas, lentils and beans act as detoxifiers. Algin, found in seaweeds, attracts lead in the gut and carries it out of the body. Yoghurt, garlic, onions, bananas and fruits such as apples and pears which contain pectin (especially the pips) help to reduce absorption, as well as detoxifying. (Spivey Fox 1975) Vitamin E may also reduce lead poisoning. (Nutrition Search Inc 1979) In animal studies sunlight has been found to help remove toxic metals. (Kime 1980)

Vitamin C, garlic, Vitamins B1 and B12 have been formulated as a cleansing tablet "Vitamin C with Garlic" by the Cantassium Company. (See Appendix one)

The FORESIGHT vitamins and minerals have been specially formulated by the FORESIGHT medical advisers for preconception, pregnancy and lactation to provide a balance of essential nutrients. These may be used in conjunction with other supplements, where need is indicated by the test results. Where doctors are in doubt, following the results of any test, FORESIGHT will be pleased to advise. The organisation has had sixteen years of experience in trace mineral supplementation to restore optimum levels and cleanse the toxic metals.

Vitamins

Fat soluble vitamins include Vitamins A, D, E, K and the essential fatty acids, sometimes called Vitamin F. Because they are fat soluble the body can accumulate stores of them against shortage even in amounts that may be toxic. However, it is rare for the body to store up so much that toxicity occurs. In industrialised countries where the diet may consist of a large amount of refined foods a person is more likely to need supplementing, especially during pregnancy.

Vitamin A

can be obtained direct from animal products in the form of retinol, or from vegetables in the form of carotene. Carotene is then changed in the body, with the help of zinc, to proplasma Vitamin A, the form the body can use, when it is needed. If sufficient zinc is not available, it is possible to become Vitamin A deficient.

Vitamin A is essential for healthy eyes, hair, skin, teeth, the mucous membranes such as the lining of the mouth, and good bone structure. It plays a part in good appetite, normal digestion, the making of red and white blood cells, and helps to make the male hormones concerned with reproduction. Deficiency problems in animals include increased susceptibility to infections, kidney stones, and reproductive system problems in both males and females. In humans the eyes are the most affected in deficiency. There are numerous reports of other conditions being helped by restored levels, such as mental illness, skin problems and sexual problems. In the animal fetus, too little Vitamin A can result in no eyes, eye defects, hydrocephalus, diaphragmatic hernia, cleft palate and cleft lip, undescended testicles, and heart defects. It is associated with neural tube defects in stillbirths.

Women with diabetes mellitus have more malformed babies than women without. Problems include microcephaly, hydrocephalus, cardiac defects, and cleft palate. Vitamin A deficiency may be involved. Vitamin A deficiency has been associated with nutritional anaemia. One study reported that, "Improvements in vitamin A status may contribute to the control of anaemic

186

pregnant women." Another study has advocated supplementing staple foods with the vitamin. However, widespread supplementation could lead to intakes that are higher than advised in some people. (Smith 1976, Smith 1973, Marks 1979, Hodges 1980, Lesser 1980, Robson 1972, Hale 1935, Jennings 1970, Davis 1954, Wald 1994, Suharno 1993)

Good Sources: Vitamin A – fish oils, especially cod liver, fatty fish, egg yolk, organ meats, whole milk, butter, cream, cheese, yoghurt.
Carotene – spinach, carrots, red pepper, broccoli, kale, chard, tomato, apricot, marrow, butter, cream.

It is best taken with full B-complex, Vitamins C, D, E, essential fatty acids, calcium, phosphorus and zinc. (Nutrition Search Inc 1979)

The Denner Report, 1990, gives 10,000iu daily as the upper limit for the supplementation of pregnant women. FORESIGHT does not give more than 5,000iu daily and usually less than this. However it should be remembered that the effects of vitiamin A deficiency on the unborn are dire. They include eye defects, hydrocephalus and genital anomalies. FORESIGHT would not advise less than 2,500iu supplementation daily.

Vitamin D

is necessary for the growth and maintenance of bones and teeth. It also aids calcium and phosphorus absorption.

Lack of Vitamin D in adults may lead to hot flushes, night sweats, leg cramps, irritability, nervousness, and depression. Other conditions include osteoporosis, osteomalacia, pains in the hips and joints, and dental caries. In children rickets and tooth decay may be present. There may be other signs of bone deformities. Poor skull development can lead to impairment of brain development. Poor jaw development may give buck teeth or snaggle teeth. It may also inhibit the function of the eustacian tubes leading to constant middle ear infection. There may be receding chins or foreheads, or large bossing foreheads with deep-set eyes. The middle face may be cramped or narrowed, pushing the palate upwards and/or forwards. Price found that most retarded children and those with learning difficulties had high raised palates. Asymmetrical development of the skull may distort the membrane carrying the blood supply to the brain cells, and inlets for the blood supply may be occluded by deformed platelets. This can affect the supply of nutrients, oxygen and glucose to the brain. Girls with insufficient Vitamin D during childhood may have narrow pelvic development which may make child birth difficult. (Marks 1979, Davis 1954, Nutrition Search Inc 1979, Lesser 1980)

Good sources: Vitamin D may be obtained in the food or through the action of the sun on the oils in the skin. This latter method is important, since food sources tend to be poor. Hence it is wise to build up stores during the summer months by allowing the action of the sun on the skin, taking precautions against sunburn.

Food sources include fish oil and fatty fish. There are small quantities in whole milk, free range eggs and butter.

It is best taken with Vitamins A and C, choline, essential fatty acids, calcium and phosphorus. (Nutrition Search Inc 1979) Liquid paraffin can prevent its absorption so should not be used. Excess Vitamin D can lead to a range of unpleasant symptoms. (Davis 1954)

Vitamin E

prevents the oxidation of Vitamin A and is needed for the utilisation of essential fatty acids and selenium. It can prevent scarring after burns, surgery and injury and is important in wound healing, such as the healing of abrasions after birth. Davis claims that some congenital heart defects will disappear if it is given from early babyhood. It has also been suggested that it has a protective effect against haemorrhage in premature babies. Researchers at the University of Edinburgh have suggested it may be another factor that can be useful in the treatment of male infertility since it is necessary for flexibility in the cell walls of the sperm – abnormal sperm are less flexible.

Without it people can develop anaemia and enlarged prostate glands. Premature aging can take place with liver and kidney damage, varicose veins and heart attacks. Phlebitis, strokes, protruding eyes, muscles degeneration and muscular dystrophy can occur.

Deficiencies in animals have caused muscular dystrophy, central nervous disorders such as encephalopathy, vascular system defects, and fetal reabsorption. In rats, deficiencies lead to abnormalities including exencephaly, hydrocephalus, joined fingers and toes and oedema. In human babies they lead to anaemia, jaundice, weak muscles, retarded heart development, brain, lung and kidney damage, backward development and squint.

Vitamin E may prevent miscarriages and helps to ease labour by strengthening muscles. Prolonged labour because of weak muscles can lead to problems for the baby as it may become starved of oxygen during the birth process. (Davis 1954, Nutrition Search Inc 1979, Tomorrow's World 1987, Williams 1973, Marks1979, Jennings 1970)

Sources: Unrefined (cold pressed) oils, whole grains, wheat germ, nuts, whole milk, egg yolk, green leafy vegetables, avocado. It is best taken with Vitamins A, full B-complex, C, essential fatty acids, manganese, selenium. (Nutrition Search Inc 1979)

Essential fatty acids (EFAs)

include, among others, linoleic, linolenic and arachidonic. They are important because they form a large part of the membranes of all cells, and they give rise to prostaglandins. These are used to make sex and adrenal hormones and affect all systems in the body. They help in the absorption of nutients and activate many enzymes. Because of the wide role of these substances in the cells, deficiencies can give rise to a large number of disorders, including allergies, gallstones, diarrhoea, varicose veins, skin problems, and heart and circulatory conditions.

In reproduction, EFA deficiency may be a factor in pre-eclampsia. There may be infertility, especially male. In rats with deficiency the pups were of lower birth weight than was expected. Deficiencies have also been reported in hyperactive children, alcoholics and drug addicts. (Horrobin 1981, Nutrition Search Inc 1979, Graham 1984, Jennings 1970, Kamen 1981)

Sources: Nuts, unrefined oils, nut butters, cold pressed oils, green leafy vegetables, seeds and fatty fish.

They are best taken with Vitamins A, C, D, E and phosphorus. (Colquhoun 1984)

Vitamin K

is generally made in the healthy intestine. It is essential for blood clotting, which explains why it is sometimes given to women in injection form at the time of birth. If the baby is short of this vitamin at birth there will be a risk of bleeding; hence it is usual to give the newly born baby an injection of it since even small haemorrhages can be serious. (Marks 1979) However, if a woman is healthy and eats plenty of green leafy vegetables she should have a good store of the vitamin and will have a baby with adequate stores.

Water soluble vitamins include the B-Complex and C. Since these are readily absorbed in water they are easily lost to the body through urine (except B12). The body does have very limited stores, though any shortage is serious.

B-Complex

B vitamins should never be taken on their own but always in conjunction with other B vitamins. Dosing with one alone may lead to a greater need for the others, thereby creating a deficiency. In nature no B vitamin is found on its own. However, it is not uncommon for a person to have a greater than usual need of any one, since we are all biochemically different. (Nutrition Search Inc 1979) (See Nutrition)

During stress, infection, pregnancy, lactation and childhood there is an increased need. Lack of almost any B vitamin leads to blood sugar problems in the body. Some of the B vitamins can be made in a healthy intestine or liver, though it is not certain how much of that synthetised can be used by the body. (Jennings 1970, Pfeiffer 1975)

B-complex is best taken with Vitamins C, E, calcium and phosphorus. (Nutrition Search Inc 1979)

Vitamin B1 (Thiamine)

is needed to break down carbohydrate into glucose. Deficiencies lead to mental symptoms such as depression, irritability, temper tantrums, failure to concentrate and poor memory. There may be fatigue, listlessness, muscle weakness, aches and pain, anorexia, neuritis, digestion problems, heart problems and shortage of breath. Deficiency in animals has been linked with sterility, relative infertility, low birth weight and stillbirth. In pregnancy it can lead indirectly to loss of appetite and vomiting, which may cause low birth weight. (Nutrition Search Inc 1979, Marks 1979, Jennings 1970, Hurley 1980, Pfeiffer 1975) Good sources : Wheat germ, rice bran, whole grains, brewer's yeast, nuts, dry beans, peas, soya beans, lentils, seeds, rice, heart, kidneys.

It is best taken with full B-complex, Vitamins C. E, manganese and sulphur. (Nutrition Search Inc 1979)

Vitamin B2 (Riboflavin)

assists in the breakdown and utilisation of carbohydrates, fats and proteins, It is essential for healthy eyes, mouth, skin, nails and hair. It works with enzymes in cell respiration.

Signs of deficiency are sensitivity to light, sore and bloodshot eyes, broken capillaries in the cheeks and nose, wrinkled or peeling lips and dry upper lips. There may be cracks at the corners of the mouth or dermatitis. Experimental animals have developed cataracts, possibly because without Vitamin B2 they could not use their Vitamin A. Since it works in conjunction with other nutrients and enzymes, deficiency symptoms may not disappear on straight supplementation with this alone.

In animal reproduction, deficiency has been found to cause sterility, stillbirths, small misshapen fetuses, reduced oxygen consumption in the liver and reduced enzyme activity. Rats have been born with blood disorders, misshapen jaws, cleft palates, joined claws, oedema, anaemia and degeneration of the kidneys. In humans, Vitamin B2 deficiency is considered to be one of the worst in pregnancy, with cleft palate and shortening of the limbs as risks. (Hodges 1980, Robertson 1962, Pfeiffer 1975, Marks 1979, Nutrition Search Inc 1979)

Sources: Brewer's yeast, liver, kidney, tongue, leafy green vegetables, whole milk, fish, butter, cheese, peas, soya beans, legumes, blackstrap molasses, egg yolks, nuts.

It is best taken with the full B-complex and Vitamin C. (Nutrition Search Inc 1979) Vitamin B2 is sensitive to light so it is destroyed if milk is left on the doorstep.

Niacin (Nicotinamide)

sometimes known as Vitamin B3 – aids in the utilisation of energy. It is important for a healthy skin, digestive system and the normal functioning of the gastrointestinal tract. It is also needed for proper nerve function, as a co-enzyme and for the synthesis of sex hormones. Deficiencies have often been linked with the three D's – dermatitis, diarrhoea and dementia. There can also be a coated tongue, mouth ulcers, anorexia, dyspepsia, diarrhoea or intermittent constipation. Mental symptoms include depression, confusion, hostility, suspicion and irrational fears. Sufferers become tense, nervous, miserable, subject to dizziness, insomnia, recurring headaches and impaired memory. Nicotinamide deficiency in rats has been found to produce cleft palate and/or hare lip and hind limb defects. (Jennings 1970, Pfeiffer 1975, Nutrition Search Inc 1979, Marks 1979, Pfeiffer 1975, Davis 1954)

Sources: Brewer's yeast, lean meats (not pork), liver, poultry, fish, wheat germ, whole grains, nuts, especially peanuts, whole milk and whole milk products. (Nutrition Search Inc 1979).

It is best taken with the full B-complex and Vitamin C.

Pantothenic acid

is needed for every cell in the body as without it sugar and fat cannot be metabolised. It is important for a healthy digestive tract, and essential for the synthesis of cholesterol, steroids and fatty acids, and the utilisation of choline and PABA. It can help the body to withstand stress. (Nutrition Search Inc 1979)

Deficiency causes a wide variety of complaints. The adrenal glands do not function, leading to a paucity of adrenal hormones which regulate balances in the body. This may cause a shortage of digestive enzymes, slow peristaltic action, indigestion and constipation following as a result. It is also linked with food allergies. As with all the B vitamins, the mental symptoms of deficiency are many, including depression, causing the sufferer to be upset, discontented and quarrelsome. There may be headaches and dizziness. These symptoms are common with low blood sugar.

In animals, deficiencies have given rise to a variety of fetal abnormalities, which mainly affect the nervous system. Cleft palate, heart defects, club foot, lack of myelination, miscarriage have been noted. Sterility is also mentioned. Similar problems in humans are also suspected. (Nutrition Search Inc 1979, Marks 1979, Williams 1973, Davis 1954, Jennings 1970)

Sources: Organ meats, brewer's yeast, egg yolks, legumes, whole grains, wheat germ, salmon, human milk, green vegetables.

It is best taken with the full B-complex, Vitamin C and sulphur. (Nutrition Search Inc 1979)

Vitamin B6 (Pyridoxine)
is needed to make use of the essential fatty acids and many of the amino acids. It is essential for growth and the synthesis of RNA and DNA. It helps maintain the balance of sodium and potassium in the body and is necessary for nerve and muscle function. It is needed for making nicotinamide in the liver. It helps prevent tooth decay, kidney stones, atherosclerosis and heart disease if it is present in abundance. Lack of B6 can mean less use is made of minerals such as zinc, magnesium and manganese There may be headaches, halitosis, lethargy, pain and cramps in the abdomen, rash around the genitals, anaemia, anorexia, nausea, vomiting, diarrhoea, haemorrhoids, dandruff, dermititis of the head, eyebrows, and behind the ears, sore lips, tongue, and a rash round the base of the nose. Hands can become cracked and sore. Night-time problems include insomnia, twitching, tremors, leg and foot cramps and bedwetting. Mental symptoms include irritability, extreme nervousness, lethargy, and inability to concentrate. Premenstrual syndrome often responds to B6 supplementation as do nausea, vomiting, oedema and the convulsions of eclampsia in pregnancy. Fetal abnormalities, including cleft palate, have been linked to B6 deficiency. Babies born with B6 deficiency have low scores on general condition ratings. There may be seizures in the new-born. (Davis 1954, Pfeiffer 1975, Williams 1973, Anon 1980b)

Sources: Meats, whole grains, organ meats, brewer's yeast, blackstrap molasses, wheat germ, legumes, peanuts.

It is best taken with full B-complex, Vitamin C, magnesium, potassium, linoleic acid and sodium. (Nutrition Search Inc 1979)

Para-amino benzoic acid (PABA)
is unique in being a "Vitamin within a vitamin". occurring in combination with folic acid. It stimulates the intestinal bacteria so they make folic acid, which is then used in the production of pantothenic acid. It helps with protein breakdown and use and in the formation of red blood cells. It is important in skin and hair colouring. It can soothe burning, especially sunburn. (Nutrition Search Inc 1979, Pfeiffer 1975)
Sources: Brewer's yeast, wheat germ, whole grains, liver and yoghurt, organ meats, green leafy vegetables.

It is best taken with full B-Complex and Vitamin C. (Nutrition Search Inc 1979)

Biotin

is necessary for the body's fat production, making fatty acids and for the oxidation of fatty acids and carbohydrates. It also helps in the utilisation of protein, folic acid, pantothenic acid and Vitamin B12. It is useful in the treatment of candidiasis.

Deficiency is linked with depression, panic attacks, extreme fatigue, muscle pain, nausea, pain around the heart, dry peeling skin, hair loss, conjunctivitis, loss of appetite, pallor of skin and mucuous membranes and lowered haemoglobin. In children there may be stunted growth and adults become thin to the point of emaciation. In rats, biotin deficiency is linked with resorption of the fetus, and death in the first few days after birth, damage to the liver, heart and blood vessels. (Nutrition search Inc 1979, Pfeiffer 1975, Chaitow 1984, Jennings 1970, Davis 1954)

Sources: Egg yolks, liver, unpolished rice, brewer's yeast, whole grains, sardines, legumes.

Raw egg white destroys biotin. It is best taken with full B-complex, Vitamin C and linoleic acid. (Nutrition Search Inc 1979)

Inositol

is needed by human liver cells and bone marrow cells. It is necessary for fat metabolism and transport, as well as healthy skin and hair. It combines with methionine and choline to make lecithin, a substance needed for the myelin sheath. Lecithin also carries Vitamins A, D, E and K around the blood.

Lack of inositol may cause falling hair, eczema, abnormalities of the eyes, constipation, irregular heart action, and a slowing down of the digestive system. (Davis 1954, Nutrition Search Inc 1979)

Sources: Whole grains, citrus fruits, brewer's yeast, molasses, meat, milk, nuts, vegetables, eggs.

It is best taken with full B-complex and linoleic acid. (Nutrition Search Inc 1979)

Choline

is needed for the formation of DNA and RNA and for making nucleic acid in the centre of the cell. It is used to make lecithin and is involved in nerve functioning. Lack of choline can lead to headaches, dizziness, strokes, haemorrage in the eye, noises in the ear, high blood pressure, awareness of heartbeat, oedema, insomnia, constipation and visual disturbances.

Because of its role in the neurotransmitter, acetylcholine, deficiency is linked with mental disorders, though its use in treatment is still under investigation. Animal experiments have shown that a lack can cause fatty liver and haemorrhages in the heart muscle and adrenal gland . It is linked with the development of stomach ulcers, liver cancer and kidney damage in young animals.

Herbicides destroy the micro-bacteria of the top-soil, preventing manganese from combining with protein. This prevents the uptake of manganese by the plants. Also organophosphates inactivate the choline containing enzymes, thus preventing manganese from crossing the gut/blood barrier, as these enzymes are needed for this. This prevents manganese getting into the blood, leading to manganese deficiency in the human. (See Minerals). (Davis 1954, Nutrition Search Inc 1979, Williams 1973, Marks 1979)

Sources: Egg yolks, organ meats, brewer's yeast, wheat germ, soya beans, fish legumes, green vegetables.

It is best taken with Vitamins A, full B-complex and Linoleic acid. (Nutrition Search Inc 1979)

Vitamin B12 (cyanocobalamin)

is needed for the production and regeneration of red blood cells, and carbohydrate, protein and fat metabolism. It helps with iron function and is used with folic acid in the synthesis of choline . It is involved in the synthesis of RNA and DNA.

Although it is often said to occur almost exclusively in animal products, this is not true. It occurs in well water that has been exposed to the soil. Dr John Douglass also reports that, "People who consume peanuts and sunflower seeds have adequate levels of B12. This indicates that the B12 is synthesised in the gut when the diet includes these foods. Eating seeds and sprouted seeds apparently provides the necessary nutrients to promote B12 synthesis."

Deficiency causes pernicious anaemia, deterioration of nervous tissue, sore mouth and tongue, neuritis, strong body odour, back stiffness, pain and menstrual disturbances and a type of brain damage. A very severe deficiency leads to deterioration of the spinal cord, with paralysis ultimately appearing.

In pregnancy the fetus does not seem to be affected by variations in the mother's level. It has been noted that if several generations of rats are kept deficient, the death rate in young animals rises sharply and their weight at four weeks is reduced. The young of deficient mothers are often hydrocephalic and have eye problems. (Pfeiffer 1975, Davis 1954, Marks 1979, Kamen1981)
Sources: Organ meats, fish and pork, eggs, milk, cheese, yoghurt. For vegetarians, useful quantities can be found in soy sauce, tempeh,miso, dulse, kelp, spirulina, seeds, sprouted seeds. Some types of brewer's yeast also contain small amounts.

It is best taken with full B-complex, Vitamin C, potassium and sodium. (Nutrition Search Inc 1979)

Folic acid

is needed for the formation of red blood cells in the bone marrow, the making of antibodies and the utilisation of sugars and amino acids. It is also important for the formation of nucleic acid, a substance essential for the growth and reproduction of all body cells, so it plays a crucial role in pregnancy. It helps the digestive processes. It works with B12 in making haemoglobin in the blood. It is essential for zinc metabolism.

Deficiency in the adult can lead to pernicious and other types of anaemia, depression, dizziness, fatigue, pallor and susceptibility to infections. Anaemia in pregnancy can be a factor in smaller placentas, urinary tract infections and premature birth. Folic acid deficiency is common, and pregnancy exacerbates it. Fetal abnormalities in the young of deficient animals include cleft palate and hare lip, deformed limbs, malformations of the heart, diaphragm, urogenital system, blood vessels, adrenals, spina bifida, malformations of the eye, skeletal deformities, underdevelopment of the lung and kidney, cataracts, brain deformities, oedema and anaemia. Fetal death and miscarriage or resorption may occur. If folic acid is given at the time of resorption the fetus may survive to term but may have hydrocephalus. If deficiency occurs during pregnancy, microcephaly can be seen in the newborn rats.

In humans, folic acid has been the subject of much attention in pregnancy, especially in the relation to neural tube defects, such as spina bifida. A number of studies have been done which suggest that women who are given supplements of folic acid in the month before conception and for the first 8-10 weeks afterwards, are less likely to have a malformed baby.

Many of the research methods of these older studies were criticised as not proving the value of folic acid supplements, and in some cases the points made were valid. However, more recent research has now lead the Government to recommend folic acid supplements for pregnant women. A year after the Government's recommendation, research in Leeds has shown that in one study of 613 women, 97.6 per cent had not increased their intake of folic acid before the critical period of fetal development. But this is not surprising given that the critical period during pregnancy when the neural tube closure in the fetus occurs is on days 26 to 27 in the embryo's life. Many women will not be aware of their pregnancy at this stage, especially if the Family Planning Association is correct in reporting that one in three babies is unplanned. The Leeds study also revealed that only 10 (1.6 per cent) of women had been prescribed or advised to take folate before conception, while one woman had been advised to eat folate rich foods.

Taking all the research into account, there can be little doubt that folate deficiency in the mother, especially in the early stages of pregnancy, can be a major contributory factor in neural tube defects. But FORESIGHT recommends that folic acid supplementation needs to be considered as part of a balanced supplementation programme. Professor Wald claimed that increasing intake by adding folate to flour used to make bread and cakes would not cause harm and would prevent 1500 of the 2000 spina bifida babies born each year. However, Pfeiffer has shown that folic acid supplementation can have adverse effects on some schizophrenics. Wholesale supplementation of the population is not advisable. Eating wholefoods which contain a balance of vitamins is preferable, with balanced supplementation as required. (See Manganese and Zinc) (Lesser 1980, Pfeiffer 1975, Kamen 1981, Jennings 1970, Dhopeshwarkar 1980, Stempak 1965, Arawaka 1967, Smithells 1980, Smithells 1987, MRC 1991, Dept Health 1992, Sutcliffe 1993, Kemble 1991, Fletcher 1994)

Sources: Green leafy vegetables, brewer's yeast, organ meats, whole grains, wheatgerm, milk, salmon, root vegetables, nuts.

It is best taken with full B-complex and linoleic acid. (Nutrition Search Inc 1979)

Vitamin C

keeps the collagen (connective tissue) healthy and resistant to penetration by viruses, poisons, toxins such as lead, dangerous drugs, allergens, and/or foreign materials. It promotes healing after surgery, infection or injury, including broken bones. It keeps the capillary walls intact. It helps the absorption of iron, preventing anaemia. It is important for mental health.

Deficiency symptoms include scurvy, dandruff, haemorrhages on the thighs, buttocks and abdomen, swollen and bleeding gums, leading to infection, ulceration and loss of teeth. There may be spontaneous bleeding. Children who are short of vitamin C are prone to infections, have poor teeth and gums. Their bones break easily, they bruise easily and quickly tire and become irritable. It has been linked with miscarriage. (Nutrition Search Inc 1979, Pfeiffer 1975, Davis 1971, Davis 1974)

Sources: Citrus fruits, rose hips, sprouted alfalfa seeds, tomatoes, green peppers, broccoli and other green vegetables, blackcurrants, strawberries and other soft fruits, bananas, apples, pears, carrot, cauliflower, new potatoes eaten with their skins, parsley. Vitamin C is lost in storage.

It is best taken with all vitamins and minerals, bioflavenoids, calcium and magnesium. (Nutrition Search Inc 1979)

APPENDIX ONE

LIST OF USEFUL ADDRESSES

Please remember to enclose SAE if
you are writing to a charity.

Action Against Allergy
24-26 High Street
Hampton Hill
Middx YW12 1PD

Active Birth Movement
52 Dartmouth Park Road
London NW5 1SL

AIMS
The Association for the Improvement
of Maternity Services
40 Kingswood Avenue
London NW6.

ALCAT
Growing Straight
Lower Broad Oak Road
West Hill, Ottery St Mary
Devon EX11 1XU

Association for Breastfeeding
Mothers
Sydenham Green Health Centre
26 Holmshaw Close
Sydenham
London SE26 4TH

ARM
Association of Radical Midwives
62 Greetby Hill
Ormskirk
Lancs L39 2DT

Biolab (mineral & medical analysis)
The Stone House
9 Weymouth Street
London W1.

British Homeopathic Association
27a Devonshire Street
London W1N 1RJ

British Society for Allergy
and Environmental Medicine
Foundation
PO Box 28
Totton
Southampton

British Society for Nutritional
Medicine
PO Box 3AP
London
W1A 3AP

Cantassium Company
Green Farm, Larkhall Grove
Laboratories
225 Putney Bridge Road
London SW15 2PY

Environmental Air Systems
Martin Wells
Sandyhill Cottage, Sandy Lane
Rushmore, Tilford,Farnham
Surrey GU10 2ET

FACT (Food Additives
Campaign Team)
25 Horsell Road
London N5 1XL

The Fertility Trust
218 Heathwood Road
Heath,
Cardiff CF4 4BS

Food Commission
third floor
5/11 Worship Street
London EC2A 2BH

FORESIGHT
28 The Paddock
Godalming
Surrey GU7 1XD

Freshwater Filters
Carlton House
Aylmer Road
Leytonstone E11 3AD

Friends of the Earth
26-28 Underwood Street
London
N1 7JQ

Good Gardeners Association
Pinetum Lodge
Churcham
Gloucester GL2 8AD

Greenpeace
30-31 Islington Green
London
N1 8XE

Healthy House
Cold Harbour
Ruscombe
Stroud Clous GL6 6DA

Henry Doubleday Research
Association
Ryton-on-Dunsmore
Coventry
Warwickshire CV8 3LG

Hyperactive Children's
Support Group
71 Whyke Lane
Chichester
Sussex

La Leche League
Spencer Lester
30 Whimbrel Way
Banbury
Oxon NW1 7YN

Maternity Alliance
59–61 Camden High Street
London NW1 7JL

McCarrison Society
c/o Institute of Brain Chemistry
and Human Nutrition,
Hackney Hospital,
Hackney Road
London, E2 8PS

National Childbirth Trust
Alexandra House
Oldham Terrace
Acton
London W3 7NH

National Society for
Research into Allergy
PO Box 45
Hinckley
Leicestershire LE10 1JY

Natural Family Planning
Mrs Colleen Norman
218 Heathwood Road
Heath,Cardiff,S Wales
Cardiff 493120 (Mornings only)

Niplette
Cannon Babysafe Ltd
Lower Road,Glenford
Sudbury
Suffolk CO10 7QS

Organic Growers Association
Aeron Park
Llangietho
Dyfed

Organic Information
PO Box 1503
Poole
Dorset BH14 8YE
01202 715130

Pesticide Exposure Group
of Sufferers (PEGS)
4 Lloyds House
Regent Terrace
Cambridge CB2 1AA

Society for Environmental Therapy
Mrs H Davidson
521 Foxhall Road
Ipswich IP3 8LW

Soil Association
86 Colston Street
Bristol BS1 5BB

Support after Termination
for Abnormalities (SAFTA)
29 Soho Square
London W1V 6JB

Toxoplasmosis Trust
61-71 Collier Street
London N1 9BE
0171-713-0663

Vitacare Ltd
The Business Centre
758–760 Great Cambridge Road
Enfield
Middlesex EN1 3RN
(for dried goats' milk)

Vitamin Service
Littlewick Road,
Lower Knaphill
Woking, Surrey (also supplies
Waymaster Crystal Water Filter)

Wholefood
(for books and organic food)
24 Paddington Street
London W1M 4DR

Wilkes and Weaver
Offa House
Offa Street
Hereford HR1 2LH
(for organic wool and cotton
mattresses)

APPENDIX TWO

FORESIGHT RECOMMENDED READING

Books

Planning for a Healthy Baby Belinda Barnes & Suzanne Gail Bradley
Studies of international research, demonstrating a variety of factors that can cause damage or ill-health in the unborn. Fortunately almost all of these can be pre-empted. The book gives the Foresight guidelines on nutrition, family planning, toxic substances to avoid and common illnesses and diseases. This gives parents the chance to give a good start to the new life by acting in time before conception takes place. £8.99 (plus 65p p&p)

The Hyperactive Child, what the family can do Belinda Barnes & Irene Colquhoun
A self-help manual written by parents of hyperactive children, explaining what hyperactivity is, what is causing it, and how they can set about dealing with the problems. £2.50 (plus 40p p&p)

Booklets

The Adverse Effects of Alcohol on Reproduction summary by Tuula Tuormaa 85p + 20p p&p

The Adverse Effects of Tobacco Smoking on Reproduction summary by Tuula Tuormaa 85p + 20p p&p

The Health Professional's Guide to Preconception Care Dr Marilyn Glenville 85p + 20p p&p

The Adverse Effects of Food Additives on Reproduction 85p +20p p&p

Find Out This little booklet has been designed to be marked up with useful notes. Additive numbers and additive names in alphabetical order are marked red for those with known adverse effects, amber for those about which there is doubt, and green for those with no known adverse effects. £1.35 + 20p p&p

Chapter from **Vitamins in Endocrine Metabolism** Isobel Jennings MRCVS, University of Cambridge. Permission was kindly given to Foresight by the author to reproduce this chapter on animal studies into causes of malformation. Available for the cost of printing (50p)

Video
Preparing for the Healthier Baby
> Foresight clinicians, researchers, voluntary workers and parents explain the Foresight philosophy and take viewers through the programme. Hire £5 per wk, or purchase price £15 + 80p p&p

Leaflets
Male Infertility (19p postage)
Natural Family Planning (19p postage)
Offers couples information on fertility awareness, teaching them to identify accurately the few fertile days in each cycle. Natural Family Planning provides an efficient means of fertility control which is non-invasive and therefore free from side-effects and health hazards.
WHY Foresight introductory leaflet (19p postage)
The Avoidance of Heavy Metals (19p postage)
The Wholefood Diet Leaflet 25p (plus 25p p&p)
The Health of the Next Generation recommneded reading for professional and lay readers (19p postage)
Preparing for Pregnancy The full Foresight programme explained (19p postage)
Six A4 posters on the Foresight philosophy and health programme (36p postage)

For further information on these and other publications, please write enclosing SAE with 29p stamp to:

Mrs Peter Barnes
Foresight
28 The Paddock
Goldalming
Surrey GU7 1XD

APPENDIX THREE

FOOD ALLERGY QUESTIONNAIRE
(JENNIFER MASEFIELD 1988)

Questionnaire for detection of food allergy

Name..

Date..

Tick in appropiate column for past/recent
symptoms. (Recent means within the last year)

		Past	Recent
Headaches	General		
	Migraine		
Face ache	Like sinusitis		
Torso and limbs	Muscular spasm		
	Weakness		
	Paralysis		
	Numbness		
	Tingling		
	Aching – localised		
	Jiggling legs		
	Restless legs		
	Shaking hands		
	Aching all over		

		Past	Recent

Arthritis
- One joint
- Many joints
- Swollen joints
- Deformed joint(s)

Eating problems
- Poor appetite
- 'Food addictions' (most favourite)
- Bingeing sessions

Irritable bowel syndrome
- Abdominal discomfort, pains
- Cramps
- Nausea
- Vomiting
- Sudden diarrhoea
- Constipation
- Lots of mucus in stool
- Belching, flatulence

Other gastrointestinal problems
- Ulcerative colitis
- Crohn's disease

Urinary problems
- Incontinence
- Late bedwetting
- Vagnitis
- Itching genital and/or rectal area

Heart
- Irregular pulse
- Palpitations
- Other?

Hyperventilation
- Fast, panting attacks
- Repeated sighing
- Repeated yawning
- Vertigo

Angioedema
- Swelling lips
- Swelling around the eyes
- Puffy face
- Swelling fingers
- Swelling ankles
- Swelling limbs
- Swelling "all over"
- Fluctuating daily weight

	Past	Recent
Asthma		
Exercise induced		
Sudden attacks		
Seasonal attacks		
During respiratory infections		

Medications

Antihistamines
Broncho-dilators
Steroids

Other

Frequent throat clearing
Recurrent cough not responding
to treatment

Rhinitis

Frequent runny nose
Seasonal runny nose
Frequent catarrh
Seasonal catarrh
Snorting noises
Itchy nose
Polyps

Conjunctivitis

Itchy watery eyes
Seasonal?
Reddened eyes
Seasonal?

Skin problems

Eczema – itchy red patches
Urticaria – nettle rash, welts
Contact dermatitis – local
itchy blisters

Scalp   Dandruff

Sensitivity   Very oversensitive to touch

Mouth problems   Scaling cracked lips
Mouth ulcers
Repeated cold sores
Geographic tongue, patchy or
spotty
Bad breath
Itchy skin after some foods

		Past	Recent

Otitis — Ear aches, repeated deafness
from fluid in ears
Bad dizziness

Psychological symptoms — Chronic fatigue
Dysrythmia
Agitation, tension, irritability
Hyperactivity
Anxiety, panic attacks
Insomnia
Short term memory loss
Stupor "coma"
Convulsions or fits, grand mal
Violent outbursts, attacks
Self-mutilation
Psychotic behaviour
Mania
True depression
Auditory hallucinations
Visual hallucinations
Depersonalisation
Separate personalities
Multiple personalities
Schizoid withdrawal

Other allergies — Insect stings where reaction
is worse than usual
Toxaemia
Animals
Feathers, birds
Paint
Drugs and medicines
Perfumes
Suspected foods
Cigarette smoke
Chemicals
Other

Allergic symptoms
in family
Mother
Father
Siblings
Grandparents

Epilepsy in family?
Mental illness in family?
Dyslexia in family?

Other comment

APPENDIX FOUR

ROTATION DIET

Monday	Tuesday	Wednesday	Thursday
Chicken	Pork	Lamb	Turkey
Banana	Sago	Brown rice	Maize(sweetcorn)
Pineapple	Dates	Rice flour	Cornflour
Beetroot	Apple	Orange	Leeks
Spinach	Pear	Grapefruit	Onions
Swiss chard	Lettuce	Satsuma	Asparagus
Pineapple juice	Endive	Mandarin	Chives
	Chicory	Lime	Grapes
	Artichoke	Carrot	Sultanas
	Snflr seeds	Celery	Grape juice
	Apple juice	Parsnip	
		Parsley	
		Orange or Grapefruit juice	

Friday	Saturday	Sunday
Fish	Rabbit	Beef
Millet	Lentils	Potato
Millet flakes	Green beans	Potato flour
Cabbage	Peas	Tomato
Savoy cabbage	Blackeyed beans	Aubergine
Brussels sprouts	Broad beans	Cucumber
Broccoli	Mung bean shoots	Marrow
Cauliflower	Plums	Melon
Kohlrabi	Peaches	Tomato juice
Swedes	Apricot	
Avocado	Cherry	
Figs	Prunes	
Water	Prune juice	

A word of warning: Withdrawal symptoms, no matter which diet is used are often associated with the removal of allergens from the diet because people are often addicted to the foods that they are allergic to. It is probably wise to start the diet when the next few days are going to be free of pressure.

If allergens are found and removed from the diet it is important to ensure that the remaining components of the diet meet the patient's nutritional requirements. Allergies may change over time or become a thing of the past if nutritional imbalances are sorted out. A person can only become really well if they deal with all their problems together, not just the allergies.

The rotation diet is designed to give each specific food only one day in seven. The diet eliminates the most common allergens, cow's milk, grains and eggs. Also, all stimulants such as coffee, tea, chocolate and the sugars. No drink should be taken except the juice of the day and water. All foods must be boiled or steamed in filtered or bottled water and plain grilled or cooked in the oven in a covered dish. No fats, oils, gravies are to be used. During the trial period NO FOOD OTHER THAN THOSE LISTED MAY BE TAKEN AT ALL.

APPENDIX FIVE

THE PATIENT'S INTRODUCTORY LETTER

Dear

I am delighted that you have booked an appointment for our preconception care clinic. The aim of the programme we are offering is to ensure that you will be in the best of health before you start your family as research has shown this will help the health of your baby, both while you are pregnant and after the birth. If you have had any problems while trying for a baby, or in a previous pregnancy, we shall investigate the possible causes. This letter gives you answers to some of the most common questions we are asked.

Do I really need to consider preconception care?
Research has shown that where the prospective parents are healthy, they have the best chance of having a healthy pregnancy and baby. This care is all the more important for those who have already had an unhappy or difficult pregnancy, a miscarriage or a baby with a problem.

What happens on the programme?
Initial appointment
Ideally we like to see both prospective parents, though if this is not possible we are happy to see one of you.
Your appointment will normally last about one hour, during which the doctor will take a medical, dietary, environmental and gynaecological history. There will also be a general medical examination. Depending on the information the doctor will then decide what tests should be done. It may mean further appointments with specialists if there are particular problems.
You will be given general advice about your diet and lifestyle as appropriate. Samples of hair may be taken for mineral/metal analysis.

Follow-up
When the tests results are known the doctor will contact you about a further appointment. At this time you will be given any necessary treatment programmes, including advice on dietary and environmental changes, and vitamin and mineral supplements required.

After a further four to five months the doctor will see you again to check on progress and make any adjustments to your programme. Other appointments will be offered as necessary.

All programmes will be discussed with patients and will be as practical as possible.

What sort of tests can I expect?

Many of the tests will be biased towards the nutritional aspects, such as hair mineral analysis. There may also be sweat mineral analysis, and blood vitamin and mineral levels looked at.

The genito-urinary and gynaecological tests ensure that there is no infection or other problem. This may involve taking a cervical swab, blood, and urine test. The man may be asked to provide a sample of blood, urine and semen if there are fertility problems.

Before you start your baby you need to be re-tested to ensure that the treatment has cleared up any problems.

How long will this take?

This depends on your health. If you need nutritional supplements then you should expect treatment to last four to six months, depending on the severity of the deficiencies. You may feel this is a long time to wait but if your body is nutritionally deficient, or has toxins such as lead, it may take at least four to five months of nutritional treatment to correct this. For the baby's sake you should be patient.

How much will it cost?

(Obviously the doctor will wish to insert his/her own costs here.)

You may wonder if you will be spending more on food and supplements. Eating a healthy diet can actually be cheaper than eating expensive but poor quality food. For example, an apple is cheaper than a bar of chocolate; wholemeal bread fills you more quickly. Fresh fruit and vegetables in season are cheaper than tinned and frozen ones.

If you smoke and/or drink you should stop and this will save you money.

As you become healthier you may also save money on drug prescriptions.

If you have further questions please ask at your consultation. Having a baby should be a wonderful experience for everyone and we want you to enjoy your preparation.

APPENDIX SIX

FORESIGHT QUESTIONNAIRE

The FORESIGHT Questionnaire is produced in leaflet form and is designed to elicit the full range of personal and enviromental factors which have a bearing on the couple's success in conceiving and delivering a healthy baby. It should be completed by both prospective parents.

It includes sections on:

the woman's previous reproductive and gynaecological history;

the man's fertility status and medical history;

contact by both partners with possible hazards.

Copies are obtainable at current printing costs from FORESIGHT.

WHOLEFOOD DIET LEAFLET

FORESIGHT believes that preconceptual nutrition is vitally important in producing healthy babies. This small leaflet sets out the dietary plan that FORESIGHT has used since 1978 to help couples planning their pregnancy.

Obtainable from:

MALE INFERTILITY LEAFLET

The research currently available directly concerned with male infertility is discussed. FORESIGHT has found that 75% of men with low sperm count have achieved fathering a child after following the FORESIGHT methods. (unpublished data, FORESIGHT 1995)

Obtainable from:

FORESIGHT
28 The Paddock
Godalming
Surrey GU7 1XD

Please send sae.

APPENDIX SEVEN

FOOD PREPARATION

Cooked or Raw food

Many famous doctors and naturopaths have advocated the benefits of raw foods, including Max Bircher-Benner, Max Gerson, Kristine Nolfi and John Douglass. Most of them recommend a diet comprising of 75 per cent raw food and 25% cooked. Why do so many of them recommend that 'cooking may damage your health'? There are many reasons quoted, only some of which we can list:

Cooking destroys vitamins. For example, if you cook fresh peas for five minutes, you destroy 20-40 per cent of Vitamin B1 and 30-40 per cent of Vitamin C.

Cooking destroys enzymes. These are essential for the efficient metabolism of food. For example, the phosphatases in milk which break down the phosphorus-containing compounds, 'are destroyed when milk is pasteurised. The result is that most of the calcium in milk contains becomes insoluble, making milk constipating.

Other proteins are deformed with some of the amino acids being destroyed, while others may be altered so they are useless.

Fats heated to high temperatures change their structure from the 'cis' type, which the body needs and uses, to the 'trans' type, which the body cannot use, and which causes harm to health.

Not all foods can be eaten raw: cooking does have some advantages.

It destroys harmful organisms, especially in meat, poultry and some shellfish. It breaks down toxins in red and black beans. It changes the tough connective tissue in meat to gelatin, making eating easier.

You can eat more cooked food than raw – maybe not an advantage if you are overweight.

Balance is the key with plenty of raw food in a varied diet.

Microwave ovens

Microwave ovens 'cook' food not by the application of heat to it, but by generating heat from within it. There is no reliable work on how cooking in microwave ovens affects the nutritional value of the food. However, we do know some of the effects of microwave energy. Regulations about leakages are strict. You may buy a detector to check for leakages but there are no standards for such devices. Some work well, others do not. It is advisable to have a qualified repairman service your oven annually.

If you must use one, do not stand near it when it is on: do not cover food with plastic to cook. We know that microwaves affect cells inside the body but we do not know the 'safe' limit of microwave exposure, though we do know that the 'safe' level has been dropping steadily over the last 20 years.

Conclusion

Knowing the contents of a healthy diet, you want to ensure that you do not spoil them by the wrong sort of preparation. A good wholefood cookbook will help, but there are some very basic guidelines.

Buy organically grown produce where possible.

Buy fresh before frozen.

Eat as much food as you can in its raw state – most vegetables and fruits are delicious raw.

Steam rather than boil.

Stir fry rather than deep fry.

Grill, roast or stew rather than fry.

Prepare food as near to eating as possible.

It is often said 'we are what we eat', and, like most cliches, there is some element of truth in it. If we want to be healthy, we must eat healthy food. If we want to have healthy children, we must recognize that this means providing the best ingredients – that is, the best food. This means food which is grown in good soil, or reared in healthy conditions, and eaten as near its natural state as possible. Fortunately, there is an increasing awareness that organic produce is superior and it is becoming more available. Enjoy it, but also recognize that with modern life-styles, it is unlikely to give you all you need to prepare for pregnancy and lactation – you will probably need to supplement it.

BIBLIOGRAPHY

Abel, Ernest L (1982) Marihuana, Tobacco, Alcohol and Reproduction, Boca
    Raton, CRC Press
Acheson, D (1989) Letter from the Chief Medical Officer on listeria in food,
    Dept Health and Social Security letter ref PL/CMo(89) 3, 16 February
Adams, MM et al (1993) Pregnancy Planning and Pre-Conception Counseling,
    Obstet Gynecol, 82 (6), 955-959
Ager, R P Oliver, R W A (1986) The Risks of Midtrimester Amniocentesis
    Biological Materials Analysis Research Unit University of Salford, 158,
    Salford, University of Salford
Airola, Paavo (1979) Every Woman's Health, Phoenix, Health Plus Publishers
Alary, Michael et al (1993) Strategy for screening pregnant women for
    chlamydial infection in a low prevalence area, Obstet Gynecol 82:399-
    404
Alder, M W (1984) ABC of Sexually Transmitted Diseases, London, BMA
Alkalay, Arie L et al (1987) Fetal varicella syndrome, J Paediat 3(3), 320-323
Allbut, T C Rolleston, H D (1906) A System of Medicine Poisonous Brews?
    The Daily Telegraph 6 October
Am J Public Health (1983)(1): 109-111
American College of Radiology (1981) Diagnostic Ultrasound in Obstetrics and
    Gynecology, Tech Bull No 63, October
Anderson, R A et al (1988) Alcohol Threat to Babies, The Sunday Times 31
    January
Andrews, L B (1984) New Conceptions, New York, St Martin's Press
Andrews, S H (1981) Abnormal reactions and their frequency in cattle
    following the use of organophosphorus warble fly dressing, The
    Veterinary Record 109: 171-175
Anke M et al (Undated) Nutritional Requirements of Nickel. Offprint available
    though FORESIGHT
Annis, L F (1978) The Child Before Birth, London, Cornell University Press
Anon (1980a) CIP Bulletin, July, St Louis
Anon (1993) Lettuce Leaks, Soil Assocation News, August
Anon (1986) Find Out, FORESIGHT
Anon (1988) Power Line Cables Link, Today, 18 March

Anon (1985) Microwaves The Invisible Danger to Expectant Mums, Healthy
    Living March: 12
Anon (1980b) The Deficiency in Vitamin B6 to Low Agpar, Medical Tribune 2
    April
Anon (1987) Boston Globe, 11 February 1987
Antonov, A N (1974) Children born during the seige of Leningrad in 1952, J
    Paediatrics 30: 250-259
Arawaka T et al (1967) Dilation of cerebral ventricles of rat offspring induced
    by 6 mercapto purine administration to dams, Tokyo J Exp Med, 91: 143
Aspock, H (Undated) Toxoplasmosis In: Prenatal and perinatal infections
    EURO reports and Studies, 93: 43-51
Atik, R B (1994) Statistics on Miscarriage, Wakefield, Miscarriage Association
Atkins, A F J Hey, E N (1991) The Northern fetal abnormality survey In: J O
    Drife and D Donnai (eds) Antenatal Diagnosis of Fetal Abnormalities,
    NewYork, Springer-Verlag
Avery, M E (1983) Born Early:The Story of a Premature Baby, Boston, Little
    Brown
Ballentine, R (1978) Diet and Nutrition, Honesdale, The Himalayan
    International Institute
Barker, D J P (1990) The fetal and infant origins of adult disease, BMJ 301;
    1111
Barlow, S M and Sullivan, F (1982) Reproductive Hazards of Industrial
    Chemicals, London, Academic Press
Barnes, B and Bradley, S G (1990) Planning for a Healthy Baby, London,
    Ebury Press
Barnes, B (1976) Hypothyroidism: The Unsuspected Illness, London, Harper
    and Row
Barrett, S (1985) Commercial Hair Analysis: Science or Scam? JAMA 25(8):
    1041-1045
Beaulac-Baillargeon, L and Desrosiers, C (1987) Caffeine-cigarette interaction
    on fetal growth, Am J Obstet Gynecol 157: 1236-1240
Becker, R (1990) Cross Currents, London, Bloomsbury
Bell, L T et al (1975) Chromosomal abnormalities in maternal and fetal tissues
    of magnesium and zinc in deficient rats, Teratology 12: 221-226
Bellinger, D et al (1987) Longitudinal analyses of prenatal and postnatal lead
    exposure and infant development in the first year, New Eng J Med 17: 1037-
    1043
Bellinger, D et al (1978) Low level lead exposure and infant development in the
    first year, Neurobehavioural Toxic and Terat 8: 151-161
Bennett, H S et al (1950) The testes, breast and prostate in men who die of
    cirrhosis of liver, Am J Clin Path 20: 814-828
Bennett, N and Neil, R (1994) The Effects of Food upon Behaviour, Nutrition
    and Crime, Nutrition and Health, 10(1):49-86
Bertell, R (1986) Mentioned in Polly Toynbee Behind the Lines, The Guardian
    15th December
Bingol, N et al (1987) Teratogenicity of cocaine in humans, J Pediatr 10(1): 93-
    96
Bithell, J F and Stewart, A M (1975) Prenatal irradiation and childhood
    malignancy: a review of British data from the Oxford survey, Br J
    Cancer 31: 271-287
Black, Sir D et al (1982) Inequalities in health: the Black Report,
    Harmondsworth, Penguin

Blackwell, A L et al (1993) Health gains from screening for infection of the lower genital tract in women attending for termination of pregnancy, Lancet 342: 206-210

Blair, J H et al(1962) MAO inhibitors and sperm production,JAMA181:192193

Blake, K D and Brown, D (1993) CHARGE association looking at the future – the voice of a family support group, Child: care, health and development, 19, 395-409

Blattner, R J (1974) The role of viruses in congenital defects, Am J Dis Child

Blumer, W R T (1980) Leaded gasoline–a cause of cancer, Envir Int 3; 465–471

Bonnell, J A (1984) Hazards In: W M Dixon and S M G Price (eds), Aspects of Occupational Health, Faber and Faber

Body, Sir R (1988) The deadly price of the farmyard antibiotic, Daily Telegraph 19th December

Brady, M See Young, Robin

Brazelton, T B (1970) Effect of Prenatal Drugs in the Behaviour of the Neonate, Am J Psychiat 126: 1296-1303

Briggs, M H (1973) Cigarette smoking and infertility in men, Med J Aust 1;616

Broadie, M (1986) Drugs and Breastfeeding, Practitioner 230: 483-485

Brook, D J H (1982) Early Diagnosis of Fetal Defects, Edinburgh, Churchill Livingstone

Brostoff, J and Gamlin, L (1989) The Complete Guide to Food Allergy and Intolerance, New York, Crown Publisher Inc

Brown, Z A (1987) Effects on infants of a first episode of genital herpes during pregnancy, N Eng J Med, 317, 1246-1251

Brunell, P A (1967) Varicella-Zoster infections in pregnancy, JAMA 199; 351-354

Bryce-Smith, D and Simpson, R I D (1984) Anorexia, Depression, and Zinc Deficiency, Lancet, ii: 1162

Bryce-Smith, D (1979) Environmental trace elements and their role in disorders of personality, intellect, behaviour and learning ability in children Proceedings of the second New Zealand Seminar on Trace Elements and Health University of Auckland, 22-26 January

Bryce-Smith, D (1981) Environmental Influences on Prenatal Development Thessaloniki Conference, September

Bryce-Smith, D and Hodgkinson, L (1986) The Zinc Solution, London, Century Arrow

Bryce-Smith D (1977) Lead and cadmium levels in stillbirths Lancet i: 1159

Brzek, A (1987) Alcohol and male fertility (Preliminary report), Andrologia 19: 32-36

Buist, R A (1984) Drug-Nutrient Interactions – An Overview, Int Clin Nut Rev 4(3)

Burcher H C and Schmidt, J G (1993) Does routine ultrasound scanning improve outcome of pregnancy? Meta-analysis of various outcome measures BMJ 307:13-17

Bushnell, P J and Bowman, R E (1977) Reversal deficits in young monkeys exposed to lead, Pharm Biochem and Behaviour 10: 733-747

Buttram, H (1994a) (Unpublished Paper)

Buttram, H (1994b) Controversial Issues -1 Candidiasis – The Phantom Illness, Unpublished paper

Caldwell D F Oberleas, D (1969) Effects of Protein and Zinc Nutrition on Behaviour in the Rat Perinatal Factors Affecting Human Development, 85: 2-8

Campbell, J M and Harrison, K L (1979) Smoking and Infertility, Med J Aust 1; 342-343

Cannon, G (1987) The Politics of Food, London, Century

Cannon, G (1983) Why Hampstead Babies are 2lbs heavier, The Sunday Times 28th March

Cannon G and Walker, C (1986) The Food Scandal, London, Century Arrow

Carlsen, E et al (1992) Evidence for decreasing quality of semen during the past 50 years BMJ 305; 609-613

Cassell, G (Ed) (1986) Ureaplasmas of humans: with emphasis on maternal and neonatal infections, Pediatric Infectious Disease 5, 6, Suppl

Catterall, R D (1981) Biological effects of sexual freedom Lancet i: 315-319

Cengiz, D et al (1991) Tackling the threat of toxoplasmosis, Midwife Health Visitor and Community Nurse, 27(7): 199-200

Chaitow, L (1984) Candida Albicans Could Yeast Be Your Problem? Wellingborough, Thorsons

Chakraborty, D et al (1978) Biochemical Studies on Polychlorinated Biphenyl Toxicity in Rats: Manipulation by Vitamin C Int J Vit Nutr Res 48: 22-31

Chan, A , Robertson, E F et al (1993) Prevalence of neural tube defects in South Australia, BMJ 307; 703-706

Chavez, G F et al (1989) Maternal cocaine use during pregnancy as a risk factor for congenital urogenital anomalies JAMA 262: 795-8

Chavkin, W (Ed)(1984) Double Exposure Women's Health Hazards – on the Job and at Home Monthly Review Press

Cherry, S H (1987) Planning Ahead for Pregnancy, London, Viking

Chitty, L S et al (1993) Effectiveness of routine ultrasonography in detecting fetal structural abnormalities in a low risk population, BMJ 303:1165-1169

Chow, W (1988) Maternal cigarette smoking and tubal pregnancy Obstet Gynecol 71: 167-174

Chrystie, I et al (1992) Screening of pregnant women for evidence of current hepatitis B infection: selective or universal? Health Trends 24(10):13-15

Churchill, JA et al (1966) Birth Weight and Intelligence, Obstet Gynecol 28: 425-9

Clausen, J and Rastogi, S C (1977) Heavy metal pollution among autoworkers 1 Lead, Br J Ind Med 34: 208-215

Colgan, M (1982) Your Personal Vitamin Profile, London, Blond and Briggs

Collins, E and Turner, G (1975) Maternal effects of regular salicylate ingestion in pregnancy Lancet ii: 335-337

Colquhoun, I and Barnes, B (1984) The Hyperactive Child What the Family Can Do, Wellingborough, Thorsons

Committee on Drugs (1983) The Transfer of Drugs and Other Chemicals into Human Breast Milk, Ped 72(3); 373-383

Consumers Associaton (1985) Drug and Therapeutics Bulletin, July 23:15

Cooper, S (1987) The Fetal Alcohol Syndrome J Child Psych and Psychiat 28: 223-227

Corbett, M and Jerrilyn, H M (1987) The Adolescent and Pregnancy, Boston, Blackwell Scientific Publications

Cott, A (1985) Help for your Learning Disabled Child The Orthomolecular Treatment, New York, Time Books

Cowdry, Q and Stokes, P (1989) Aluminium causes senility The Daily Telegraph, 13 January

Crane, M J (1992) The diagnosis and management of maternal and congenital syphilis, J Nurse Midwif 37(1): 4-16

Crawford, I L and Connor, J D (1975) Zinc and Hippocampal Function, J Orthomol Psych 4(1): 39-52

Crook, W G (1983) The Yeast Connection, Professional Books

Crosby, W M et al (1977) Fetal Malnutrition: An Appraisal of Correlated Factors, Am J Obstet Gynaecol 128: 26

Crosby, W M et al (1977) Fetal malnutrition: an appraisal of correlated factors, Am J Obstet Gynecol 128: 22

Crum, L A and Fowlkes, J B (1986) Acoustic cavitation generated by microsecond pulses of ultrasound, Nature 319 2 January

Dahle, A J et al (1970) Progressive hearing impairment in children with congenital cytomegalovirus infection, J Speech Hear Dis 44: 220

Dankenbring, WF (1974) Your Keys to Radiant Health, New Canaan, KeatsPub

David, O J et al (1976) Lead and hyperactivity Behavioural response to chelation: a pilot study, Am J Psychiat 133(10): 1155-1158

Davies, S (1981) Lead, Beyond Nutrition, Summer 12-13

Davies, S and Stewart, A (1987) Nutritional Medicine, London, Pan

Davis, A (1974) Let's have healthy children, Unwin Paperbacks

Davis, A (1954) Let's Eat Right to Keep Fit, New York, New American Library

Davis, D R (1981) Wheat and Nutrition, Nutrition Today 16(4)

Davis, J et al (1966) Effects of phenelzine on semen in infertility: a preliminary report, Fert Ster 17: 221-225

De Matteo (1985) The Terminal Shock, Toronto, NC Press

Department of Health (1992) Folic acid and the prevention of neural tube defects: report from an expert advisory group, Heywood: Do H Health Publication Unit

Department of Health (1994) Report on confidential enquiries into maternal deaths in the United Kingdom 1988 – 1990, London, HMSO

Dhopeshwarkar, G A (1980) Nutritional and Brain Development, New York, Plenum Press

Dispatches (1988) Channel 4, 8 January

Dispatches (1995) Channel 4, "Chorion Villus Sampling", 15th March

Dixit, V P et al (1983) Effects of a single ethanol injection into the vas deferens on the testicular function in rats, Endrokrinologie 67: 8-13

Dixon, H G (1980) Obstetrics and Gynaecology, London, Wright

Dohen, S R and Thompson, J W (1990) Otitic candidiasis in children: an evaluation of the problem and effectiveness of ketaconazole in 10 patients, Ann Otol Rhinol Laryngol 99: 427-431

Dougherty, Ralph In: Anon Unplugging the Gene Pool, Outside, September 1980: 13

Douglas, C P (1984) In: G Chamberlain,(ed) Contemporary Obstetrics, London, Butterworths

Doyle, W et al (1990) The association of maternal diet and birth dimensions, J Nut Med 1: 7-9

Drife, J (1994) The case for sterilisation, The Times 20 December

Duffy, F H et al (1979) Long-Term Effects of an Organophosphate upon the Human Electroencephalogram, Toxicology and Applied Pharmacology 47; 161-176

Duffy, F H and Burchfield, J L (1980) Long Term Effects of the Organophosphate Sarin in EEGs in Monkeys and Humans, Neurotoxicology 1: 667-689

Dulfer, S (1987) Hepatitis B and the newborn a case for vaccination, Maternal and Child Health 12: 206-212

Eagle, R (1986) Eating and Allergy, Wellingborough, Thorsons

Eberhart-Philips, J E et al (1993) Measles in pregnancy: a descriptive study of 58 cases, Obstet Gynaecol 82: 797-801

Ebrahim, G J (1979) The Problems of Undernutrition In: Ed: R J Jarrett Nutrition and Disease, Baltimore, University Park Press

Editorial (1964) The Drugged Sperm BMJ 1: 1063-1064

Edwards, M J (1967) Congenital defects in guinea pigs following induced hyperthermia during gestation, Arch of Pathology, 84: 42-48

Eilard, T et al (1976) Isolation of chlamydia in acute salpingitis, Scand J Infectious Dis (Suppl 9), 82-84

El-Dakhakny, A and El-sadik, Y M (1972) Lead in hair among exposed workers, Am Ind Hygiene Assoc Journal 33

Elam, D (1980) Building Better Babies Preconception Planning for Healthier Children, Millbare, Celestial Arts

Elek, S D and Stern, H (1974) Development of a vaccine against mental retardation caused by cytomegalovirus infection in utero, Adv Teratology 4: 62

Elkington, J (1985) The Poisoned Womb, Harmondsworth, Viking

Erdmann, R (1987) The Amino Revolution, London, Century Paperbacks

Erlichman, J (1993) Sheep dip alarm likely to force ban, The Guardian 26 October

Erlichman, J (1986) Gluttons for Punishment, London, Penguin

Evans, H J et al, (1981) Sperm abnormalities and cigarette smoking, Lancet, i: 627-629

Fantel, A G and Macphail, B J (1982) The teratogenicity of cocaine, Teratology 26: 17-19

Fedrick, J and Anderson, A (1976) Factors associated with sponateous pre-term birth, Br J Obstet Gynaecol 83: 342

Ferreira, A J (1969) Prenatal Environment, Springfield, Charles C Thomas

Fine, P E M et al (1985) Infectious diseases during pregnancy: a follow-up study of the long-term effects of exposure to viral infections in utero, London, HMSO

Finkel, M J (1979) National foundation/March of Dimes Symposium on Drug and chemical risks to the fetus and new born infant, NY City, 21 May

Firth, H V et al (1994) Analysis of limb reduction defects in babies exposed to chorionic villus sampling, Lancet, 343: 1069-1071

Fletcher, D (1988) Scourge of the Sick Building Syndrome, Daily Telegraph 24 March

Fletcher, D (1994) Cake recipe may prevent spina bifida, Daily Telegraph, 13th January

Fletcher, D (1988) Pregnant Women being Sought for Trials with Aspirin, Daily Telegraph 29 August

Fletcher, D J (1982) Hair Analysis Proven and problematic applications, Postgrad Med 72(5): 79-88

Fox, M (1994a) Green Network Briefing – Oestrogen Mimics, Green Network Briefing, March, Green Network

Fox, M (1994b) Green Network Briefing – Oestrogen Mimics, Green Network Briefing, May, Green Network

Fox, M (1994c) Green Network Briefing – Oestrogen Mimics, Green Network Briefing, June, Green Network

Franc, M C , Meunier, A et al (1981) Archives du Malades Professionnelles, du Medicin du Travail et du Securite Sociale, 42(3): 183-194

Frank, C (1994) Caesarean births, The Times, 12 December

Freundlich, M et al (1985) Infant Formula as a Cause of Aluminium Toxicity in Neonatal Ureamia, Lancet ii: 527-529

Friberg, J and Gnarpe, H (1973) Mycoplasma and human reproductive failure, Am J Obstet Gynecol, 116: 23-26

Friend, J (1994) Caesarean births, The Times, 23 December

Froas, J et al (1993) Fetal exsanguination by chorion villus sampling, Lancet 342:1159

Fromell, G T et al (1979) Chlamydial infections of mothers and their infants, J Ped 95(1):28-32

Furuhashi, N et al (1985) Effects of Caffeine Ingestion During Pregnancy, Gynecol Obstet Investigation 19: 187-191

Gal, I et al (1967) Hormonal prengancy tests and congenital malformations, Nature 216:83

Gardner, N and Nuki, P (1994) Solvent may hurt unborn, The Sunday Times 4 September

Garnys, V et al (1979) Lead Burden of Sydney Schoolchildren, University of New South Wales

Gellin, B G B and Brume, C V (1989) Listeriosis, JAMA 261:1313-1319

Gennser, G et al (1988) Low birth weight and risk of high blood pressure in adulthood, BMJ 296; 1498-1500

Gibbs, C E and Seitchik, J (1980) Nutrition in Pregnancy In: R S Goodhart and M Shils (eds) Modern Nutrition in Health and Disease, Philadephia, Lea and Febiger

Gibbs, R S (1987) Microbiology of the female genital tract, Am J Obstet and Gynecol 156:491-495

Gill, L (1992) A fertile area of anxiety for the male, TheTimes 22 May

Gittelman, R and Eskenazi, B (1983) Lead and hyperactivity revisited, Arch Gen Psychiat 40: 827-833

Glenville, M (Undated) Health Professionals' Guide to Preconception Care, FORESIGHT, Godalming

Goldenburg, R L et al (1993) Pregnancy Outcome Following a Second-Trimester Loss, Obstet and Gynecol, 81: 444-446

Goldhaber, M K et al (1988) Am J Industrial Medicine 13: 695

Gordon, G F (1980) Hair Analysis: Its Current Use and Limitations Part II, Let's Live, October: 89-94

Goujard, J et al (1978) Maternal Smoking and Alcohol Consumption and Abruptio Placentae, Am J Obstet Gynecol 130: 738

Graham, J (1984) Evening Primrose Oil, Wellingborough, Thorsons

Grant, E C G (1979) Food Allergies and Migraine, Lancet i; 966-968

Grant, E (1985) The Bitter Pill, London, Corgi

Grant, E (1988) Personal communication April

Grant, E (1986) The Effect of Smoking on Pregnancy and Children In: Guidelines for Future Parents, FORESIGHT

Grant, E (1994) Sexual Chemistry: Understanding our Hormones, the Pill and HRT, London, Cedar

Gray's Anatomy (1954)

Gray, J A (1990) Orchitis in chicken pox Br J Gen Practice December: 522

Green, J and Statham, H (1993) Testing for fetal abnormality in routine antenatal care Midwifery, 9: 124-135

221

Greenhalgh, T (1995a) Scourge of women in the West, The Times 10 January

Greenhalgh, T (1995b) Will a pill a day keep clots at bay? The Times 31January

Gullen, M T et al (1990) Transvaginal ultrasonographic deletion of congenital abnormalities in the first trimester, Am J Obstet and Gynecol 163(2): 446-476

Haire, D (1983) Fetal Effects of Ultrasound: A Growing Controversy, Int Soc Psychosomatic Obstet Gyn 7th International Congress, September 14-15

Hale, F (1935) Pigs born without eye balls, J Hered,24: 105-106

Hall, M (1988) The Agony and the Ecstacy, Channel Four, 14 April

Hambidge, K M et al (1972) Low Levels of Zinc in Hair, Anorexia, Poor Growth, and Hypogeusia in Children, Pediat Res, 6: 868-874

Hansen, J C et al (1980) Children with minimal brain dysfunction, Danish Med Bull 27(6): 259-262

Hanshaw, J B (1970) Developmental abnormalities associated with congenital cytomegalovirus infection Adv Teratology 4: 62

Hardy, P H et al (1984) Prevalence of six sexually transmitted disease agents among pregnant inner-city adolescents and pregnancy outcome Lancet ii:333-337

Harlap, S et al (1985) Congenital Abnormalities in the Offspring of Women Who Used Oral and Other Contraceptives Around the Time of Conception Int J Fert 30: 39-47

Harris, R and Read, A P (1981) New Uncertainties in Pre-natal Screening for Neural Tube Defect BMJ 282: 1416-1418

Harrison, L (1990) Making Fats and Oils Work for You, New York, Avery Publishing Group Inc

Hawkes, N (1994a) Struggling sperm's clue to infertility, The Times 22 December

Hawkes, N (1994b) Doctors find added risk for Pill users, The Times 25 November

Hawkes, N (1994c) Should you worry about the Pill? The Times 17 May

Hawkes, N (1994d) Babies may be paying a high price for grandmother's habit, The Times 3 February

Hay, M (1989) Neonatal listeriosis and ventriculomegaly: Two case reports, Mat and Child Health 14 (1): 14-15

Hay, P et al (1994) Abnormal bacterial colonisation of the genital tract and subsequent preterm delivery and late miscarriage, BMJ 308: 295-8

Health Education Council (1983) A discussion paper on proposals for nutritional guide lines for health education in Britain Prepared for the National Advisory Committee on Nutrition Education by an ad hoc working party under the Chairmanship of Professor V P T James, London, NACNE

Health Education Council (1985) Herpes: What It is and How To Cope, London, HEC

Hellstrom, B et al (1976) Prenatal sex-hormone exposure and congenital limb reduction anomalies, Lancet ii; 372-373

Henry-Suchal et al (1980) Microbiology of specimens obtained by laparoscopy from controls and from patients with pelvic inflammatory disease or infertility with tubal obstruction, chlamydia trachomatis, ureaplasma urealyticum, Am J Obstet Gynaecol 138: 1022

Himmelberger, D U et al (1978) Cigarette smoking during pregnancy and the occurrence of spontaneous abortion and congenital abnormality, A J Epid 108: 470-479

Hodges, R E and Adelman, R D (1980) Nutrition in Medical Practice, Philadelphia, W B Saunders

Hoffer, A (1983) Orthomolecular Nutrition at the Zoo, Orthomolecular Psychiatry 12(2): 116-128

Holiverda-Kuipers, J (1987) The cognitive development of low birthweight children, J Child Psych and Psychiat 28: 321-8

Hollingworth, B et al (1987) Colposcopy of women with cervical HPV type 16 infection but normal cytology, Lancet ii: 1148

Hornsby, M (1993) Insecticide might be "mad cow" link, The Times, 21st August

Horrobin, D F (1981a) The Importance of Gamma-Linolenic Acid and Prostaglandin E1 in Human Nutrition and Medicine, J Holistic Med 3(2): 118-139

Horrobin, D (1981b) See Kamen, Betty and Si below

HSA Toxicity Review A195-645 (Undated) London, HMSO

HSA Toxicity Review: Toluene (Undated) London, HMSO

Huisjes, H J (1984) Spontaneous Abortion In: Current Reviews in Obstetrics and Gynaecology, Edinburgh, Churchill Livingstone

Hurley, L (1980) Developmental Nutrition, Englewood Cliffs, New Jersey, Prentice-Hall

Hurley, L S et al (1976) Teratogenic effects of magnesium deficiency, J Nut 106: 1254-1260

Hurley, L (1969) Zinc Deficiency in the Developing Rat, Am J Clin Nut 22: 1332-1339

Irvine, D S (1994) Falling sperm quality, BMJ, 309: 476

Israel, K S et al (1975) Neonatal and childhood gonococcal infections, Clin Obs Gyn 18: 143-151

Jacob, M et al (1987) A forgotten factor in pelvic inflammatory disease: infection in the male partner, BMJ: 294: 869

Jameson, S (1984) Zinc Status and Human Reproduction In; Zinc in Human Medicine Proceedings of a Symposium on the role of Zinc in Health and Disease, Isleworth, TIL Publications Ltd

Janerich, D T et al (1974) Oral contraceptives and congenital limb reduction defects New Eng J Med 291(ii): 696-700

Jennings, I W (1970) Vitamins in Endocrine Metabolism, London, Heinemann

Jervis, R and N (1984) The FORESIGHT Wholefood Cookbook, London, Roberts Publications

Joffe, J M (1979) Influence of Drug Exposure of the Father on Perinatal Outcome, Clinics in Perinatology, Symposium of Pharmacology, 6(1): 21-36

Johnson, A et al (1993) Functional abilities at age 4 years of children born before 29 weeks of gestation BMJ 306: 1715-1718

Johnson, M K (1975) The Delayed Neuropathy Caused by Some Organophosphorus Esters: Mechanism and Challenge, Critical Reviews in Toxicology, June 289: 313

Judges, 13: 3-4

Kamen, B and S (1981) The Kamen Plan for Total Nutrition During Pregnancy, New York, Appleton-Century-Croft (This is an excellent book)

Kaufman, M In: Neville Hodgkinson, Alcohol Threat to Babies, The Sunday Times 31 January

Kays, C (1984) The RCGP's Oral Contraceptive Study: Some Recent Observations Clinics in Obstetrics and Gynaecology, 11:3

Keller Phelps, J and Norse, A (1986) The Hidden Addiction and How To Get Free, Boston, Little Brown and Company (An excellent "How To" book)

Kemble, B (1991) Why one baby in three is a surprise Evening Standard 12Nov

Kilham, L and Ferm, V H (1976) Exencephaly in fetal hamsters following exposure to hyperthermia, Terat, 14: 323-326

Kime, Z R (1980) Sunlight, Penryn, World Health Publications

Kirk, K M and Lyon, M F (1984) Induction of congenital malformations in the offspring of male mice treated with pre-meiotic and post-meiotic stages, Mutation Research '125: 75-85

Klevay, L M (1978) Hair as a Biopsy Material Progress and Prospects, Arch Intern Med 138: 1127-1128

Kostial, K and Kello, D (1979) Bioavailability of lead in rats fed "human diets", Bull Environ Contam Toxic 21: 312-314

Kricker, A et al (1986) Congenital limb reduction deformities and use of oral contraceptives Am J Obstet Gynecol 155: 1072-1078

Kucheria, K et al (1985) Semen analysis in alcohol dependence syndrome, Andrologia 17: 558-563

Kulikauskas, V et al (1985) Cigarette smoking and its possible effects on sperm, Fert Ster 44: 526-528

Kupsinel, R Mercury Amalgam Toxicity A Major Common Denominator of Degenerative Disease, J Orthomolecular Psychiat 13(4): 240-257

Labadarios, D (1975) Studies on the Effects of Drugs on Nutritional Status PhD Thesis, University of Surrey, Guildford

Lacranjan, I (1975) Reproductive ability of workmen occupationally exposed to lead, Arch Envir Health 20: 396-401

Laker, M (1982) On determining trace element levels in man: the uses of blood and hair Lancet ii: 260-262

Lancet (1983) Food Allergy: How Much is in the Mind, Lancet i: 1259-1261

Lancet (1985) Editorial 9 November

Lancet(1987) ii: 1153

Lappe, M (See Lodge Rees)

Laurance, J, (1992) Global sperm counts have almost halved in the past 50 years, The Times 11 September

Laurance J (1994) Childbirth trust seeks inquiry into varied Caesarean rates, The Times 6 December

Laurence, K M et al (1980) Increased risk of recurrence of neural tube defects to mothers on poor diets and the possible benefits of dietary counselling, BMJ 281: 1509-1511

Lazebik, N et al (1988) Zinc Status, Pregnancy Complications and labor, Abnormalities, Am J Obstet Gynecol, 158: 161-166

Leck, I (1978) Maternal hyperthermia and anencephaly, Lancet i: 671-672

Lesser, M (1980) Nutrition and Vitamin Therapy, New York, Bantam

Lester, M L et al (1986) Protective Effects of Zinc and Calcium Against Heavy Metal Impairment of Children's Cognitive Function, 145-161

Levy, E P et al (1973) Hormone treatment during pregnancy and congenital heart defects, Lancet, i:611

Lightfood, L and Rogers, L (1995) Hundreds killed by doctors relying on outdated manuals, The Times, 5 February

Lindsay S et al (1993) Interactions of human immunodeficiency virus infection and pregnancy, Obstet Gynaecol, 82: 787-796

Lin-Fu, J S (1973) Vulnerability of children to lead exposure and toxicity, New Eng J Med 289: 129-1233

Lipsett, M B (1980) Physiology and pathology of the Leydig cell In: M C
    Bleich, M J Moore (eds) Seminars in Medicine, New Eng J Med 85:
    682-688
Little, R E and Sing, C F (1987) Father's Drinking and Infant Birth Weight:
    Report of an Association, Terat, 36;59-65
Lodge Rees, E (1983) Trace elements in pregnancy In: J Rose (Ed) Trace
    Elements in Health, London, Butterworths
Lodge Rees, E (1981) The concept of preconceptual care, Intern J Envir Studies
    17: 37-42
Lodge Rees, E (1983) Prevention versus problems in pediatric science In: The
    Next Generation, FORESIGHT
Lodge Rees, E (1979) Aluminium Toxicity as Indicated by Hair Analysis,
    J Orthomol Psychiat 8(1): 137-143
Lumley, H (1992) In: Horizon, BBC2, A Diet for a Lifetime
Lya den Ouden, A et al (1993) School performance in very preterm children,
    Lancet 342; 28 August
MAFF (1994a) Personal Communication 17 February
MAFF (1994b) Personal Communication 8 March
Magenis, P G et al (1977) Parental origin of the extra chromosome in Down's
    syndrome, Human Genetics, 37: 7-16
Mahalik, M P et al (1980) Teratogenic potential of cocaine hydrochloride in
    CF-1 mice, J Pharm Sci, 69: 703-706
Mann, P (1985) Marijuana Alert, New York, McGraw-Hill
Mansfield, P and Munro, J (1987) Chemical Children, London, Century
Marcovitch, H (1994) Babies on a borderline, The Times 12 April
Mardh, P H (1981a) Medical chlamydiology: A position paper, Scan J Infect
    Dis (Supp 32):3-8
Mardh, P H et al (1981b) Endometriosis caused by chlamydia trachomatis, Br J
    Vene Dis, 57-91
Marks, J (1979) A Guide to the Vitamins, Lancaster, Medical and Technical
    Publishers Company Ltd
Masefield, J (1988) Psychiatric Illness caused or exacerbated by Food Allergies
    (Unpublished article)
Masters, W H and Johnson, V E (1970) Human Sexual Adequacy, Boston,
    Little, Brown and Company
Mastroiacovo, P (1995) In Dispatches
Mau, G and Netter, P (1974) Deutsche Medizinische Wochenschrift, 99; 1113-
    1118
Maugh, T H (1978) Hair: A Diagnostic Tool to Complement Blood Serum and
    Urine, Science 202: 1271-1273
May, D (1992) Some Substances Known or Suspected of harming Male
    Reproductive Health of Their Offspring, Midsummer Newsletter,
    Godalming, FORESIGHT
May, P A et al (1991) Epidemiology of fetal alcohol syndrome among
    American Indians of the southwest, Social biol, 30: 374-387
McCarrison, Sir R (1984) Nutrition and Health, London, McCarrison Society
McCarthy, P (1988) Health, February
McCredie, J et al (1984) Congenital Limb Defects and the Pill, Lancet, ii; 623
McCree, D In: M Gold Additional findings at low exposures have prompted
    serious second thoughts about US safeguards, Science 80 Prem issue, 81
McEwan, J (1986) Contraceptive Sponges, Maternal And Child Health,
    October, 336-341

McGee, R and Stanton, W R (1994) Smoking in pregnancy and child development to age 9 years , J Paediat 30; 263-268

McKie, R, (1983) Cadmium in the diet poses health danger The Sunday Times, 25 September

McNay, M B (1987) Diagnostic ultrasonography, Clin Obstet and Gyncaecol, 1:1

Medical Research Council Working Party on Amniocentesis (1978) An Assessment of the Hazards of Aminocentesis, Br J Obstet Gynaecol, 85, suppl 2, 1-41

Medical Research Council Vitamin Study Group (1991) Prevention of neural tube defects: results of the Medical Research Council vitamin study, Lancet, i: 338: 131-137

Mendelsohn, A (1985) (See Mann, P)

Micic, S et al (1990) Seminal Antisperm Antibodies and Genitourinary Infection Urology, XXXV (1): 54-56

Mill and Sutton, G (1979) J Antibiotics, 32(9), 915-919

Miller, H C et al (1976) Am J Obstet Gynaecol, 125; 55-60

Millstone, E & Abraham, J (1988) Additives A Guide for Everyone, Penguin

Minkoff, H et al (1987) Aids related complex: Follow up of mothers, children and subsequently born siblings, Obstet Gynecol, 69: 288-291

Mohsen Moussa, M (1983) Caffeine and sperm motility, Fert Ster, 39: 845-848

Montagu, A (1961) Life Before Birth, New York, New American Library

Moore, D E et al (1980) Association of chlamydia trachomatis with tubal infertility, Fert Ster,34: 303-304

Moore Lappe, F (1975) Diet for a Small Planet, New York, Ballentine

Moore, L S and Fleischman, A (1975) Subclinical Lead Toxicity, Orthomol Psychiatry 4(1): 61-70

Morris, MKG and Hill, CS (1992) Assessing congenital heart defects in the cocaine-exposed neonate, Dimensions of Critical Care Nursing, 11(1)

Mortensen, M L et al (1986) Teratology and the Epidemiology of Birth Defects In: S G Gabbe et al (Eds) Obstetrics Normal and Problem Pregnancies, New York, Churchill Livingstone

Mortimer, G R (1975) In the Beginning: Your Baby's Brain Before Birth, New York, New American Library

Mulvihill, J J et al (1990) Congenital Heart Defects and Prenatal Sex Hormones, Lancet i; 1168

Munday, P E (1983) Chlamydial infection In: Progress in Obstetrics and Gynaecology 3; 231-245

Murray, P et al (1990) Medical Microbiology, London, Wolfe Pub Ltd

Myhill, S Enzyme Potentiated Desensitisation Paper delivered at FORESIGHT conference in December 1991

Naeye, R L and Peters, E D (1982) Work during pregnancy effects the fetus, Pediatrics 69: 724-7

Naeye, R L (1979) JAMA, 241

Nance, S (1982) Premature Babies, Arbour House

National Center for Devices and Radiological Health of the Food and Drug Administration of USA (1982) FDA Pub No 82-8190

Naylor, G J et al (1984) Elevated Vanadium Content of Hair and Mania, Biol Psych 19(5): 759-763

Needleman, H L et al (1979) Deficits in psychologic and classroom performance of children with elevated dentine lead levels, New Eng J Med 300: 689-696

Needleman, H L et al (1990) New Eng J Med 332: 83-88

Needleman, H L et al (1984) JAMA 251(22): 2956-9

Nevison, J (1993) Unpublished paper Details available through FORESIGHT

Ng, T P et al (1992) Risk of Spontaneous Abortion in Workers Exposed to Toluene, Br J Indust Med, 49(11): 804-809

Nicholas, N S (1990) Urinary tract infections in pregnancy, Mat and Child Health, October 294-297

Nieburg, P et al (1985) The Fetal Alcohol Syndrome, JAMA, 253: 2998-2999

Nielson, F H (1984a) Nickel In: Earl Frieden, (Ed) Biochemistry of the Essential Ultratrace Elements, Plenum Publishing

Nielson, F H (1984b) Fluoride, Vanadium, Nickel, Arsenic, and Silicon in Total Parental Nutrition, Bull of the New York Academy of Med, 60(2), 177-195

Nikolaides, K (1995) In Dispatches, (1995) above

Nomura, T (1982) Parental exposure to X rays and chemicals induces heritable tumours and anomalies in mice, Nature 296; 575-577

Nora, A and Nora, J J (1975) A Syndrome of Multiple Congenital Anomalies Associated with Teratogenic Exposure, Arch Envir Health, 30: 17-21

Nora, J J et al (1978) Exogenous progestogen and estrogen implicated in birth defects, JAMA, 240(9), 837

Nordstrom, S et al (1981) Reproductive hazards among workers at high-voltage systems, Bioelectromagnetics, 4: 91-101

Nordstrom, S et al (1983) Genetic defects in offspring of power-frequency workers, Bioelectromagnetics, 4: 91

Noritoshi, T et al (1994) Prenatal exposure to influenza and the development of schizophrenia: is the effect confined to females? Am J Psychiat 151: 1127-1129

Norwood, C (1980) At Highest Risk, New York, McGraw-Hill

Nutrition Search Inc (1979) Nutrition Almanac, New York, McGraw-Hill

Nuttall, N (1994a) Crisp bags linked to male infertility, The Times 25 October

Nuttall, N (1994b) Household detergents 'may wash away male virility', The Times 9 September

Nuttall, N (1994c) Government urged to cut benzene levels, The Times 3 February

Nuttall, N (1994d) Diseased fish found in water supply, The Times 12 October

Oakley, G P et al (1973) Hormonal pregnancy tests and congenital malformations, Lancet ii: 256-257

Oberleas, D et al (1972) Trace Elements and Behaviour, Int Review Neurobiology Sup

Onwudiegwu, U and Bako, A (1993) Male contribution to infertility in Nigerian community, J Obstet Gynaec 13: 135-138

Ostrea, E M and Chaves, C J (1979) Perinatal problems (excluding neonatal withdrawal) in maternal drug addiction: a study of 830 cases, J Pediat, 94: 292-295

OPCS Monitor (1984) Reference DH3 84/2 Issued 1 May

OPCS Monitor (1987) Reference MB3 87/1 Issued 22 September

OPCS (1991a) Mortality Statistics Perinatal and Infant Series DS3

OPCS (1991b) Congenital Malformations Statistics Notifications MB3

Ortho-Cilag, (1987) ORTHO-NOVIN* 1/50 Oral Contraceptive Tablets, High Wycombe, Ortho-Cilag Pharmaceutical Limited

Ott, J N (1985) Light, Radiation and You, Greenwich,

Pallot, P (1990) Drug warning on infertility, The Times, 28 November

Parker, K et al (1991) Diagnostic Amniocentesis before 16 weeks, J Obstet Gynaecol, 11: 109-111

Passwater, R (1980) Selenium as a Food Medicine, New Canaan, Keats Publishing Co

Passwater, R and Cranton, E (1983) Trace Elements, Hair Analysis and Nutrition New Canaan, Keats Publishing Co

Pauling, L (1971) The significance of the evidence about ascorbic acid and the common cold, Proc Nat Acad Sci, 68: 2678-2681

Pfeiffer, C C (1975) Mental and Elemental Nutrients New Canaan, Keats Publishing Co

Pfeiffer, C C (1978) Zinc and Other Micronutrients New Canaan, Keats Publishing Co

Pharoach, P O D et al (1971) Neurological damage to the fetus resutling from severe iodine deficiency during pregnancy Lancet i: 308-310

Phil, R O and Parkes, M (1977) Hair element content in learning disabled children Science 198: 4214

Pitkin, R M et al (1972) Maternal Nutrition, A Selective Review of Clinical Topics Obstet Gynaecol 40: 775

Plant, M (1987) Reported in K Gill Alcohol "Safe in Pregnancy?" The Times 4 November

Polakoff, P (1984) Work and Health It's Your Life Washington, Press Assoc Inc

Pottenger, F M (1983) Pottenger's Cats La Mesa, Price-Pottenger Foundation

Prentice, T (1988) Anguish of the Sterile Husbands The Times 20 April

Prentice, T (1990) Heart Attack Risk linked to lack of foetal growth, The Times, 3 August

Price, W A (1945) Nutrition and Physical Degeneration, La Mesa, Price-Pottenger Foundation

Public Eye (1995) Little Miracles BBC2 31st January

Purdey, M (1988) Personal communication

Pyktowitx Streissguth, A (1987) Aspirin and Acetaminophen Use by Pregnant Women and Subsequent Child IQ and Attention Decrements, Terat, 35:211-219

Ramsey Tainsh, A (1984) Mycotoxicosis and Birth Defects, Paper given in May

Rantala, M L and Korkimies, A I (1986) Semen quality of infertile couples – comparison between smokers and non-smokers Andrologia 19: 42-46

Reading, R et al (1993) Deprivation, low birth weight, and children's heights: a comparison between rural and urban areas BMJ 307: 1458-1462

Reading, C and Meilon, R (1984) Relatively Speaking Sydney, Fontana

Reusens, B et al (1979) Controlling Factors of Fetal Nutrition In: Carbohydrate Metabolism in Pregnancy Ed Sutherland, H V

Rhodes, A J (1961) Virus and Congenital Malformations: Papers and Discussions presented at the First International Conference on Congenital Malformations, Philadelphia-Lippincott

Ridge, B R and Budd, G M (1990) How long is too long in a spa pool? New Eng J Med 323: 835-836

Ritchie, J W K and Thompson, W (1982) A Critical Review of Amniocentesis in Clinical Practice In: J Bonner (Ed) Recent Advances in Obstetrics and Gynaecology, Edinburgh, Churchill-Livingstone

Robaire, B and Hales, B F (1993) Paternal exposure to chemicals before conception, BMJ, 307; 341-342

Roberts, D (Undated) Pharmacology and toxicology of organophosphorus pesticides, Offprint available from FORESIGHT

Robertson, WF (1962) Thalidomide (Distival) and vitamin B deficiency BMJ1: 792

Robson, JRK (1972) Malnutrition: its causation and control New York, Gordon and Breach

Rodriguez, A F et al (1986) Relationship between benzodiazepine ingestion during pregnancy and oral clefts in the newborn, a case-control study, Med Clin 87/18: 741-743

Rogers, L and Lightfoot, L (1994) Women die as childbirth guidelines are ignored, The Sunday Times, 16 October

Rose, J Ed: (1983) Trace Elements in Health London, Butterworths

Rosenthal, N et al (1985) Antidepressant Effects of Light in Seasonal Affective Disorder Am J Psychiat 2; 163-170

Rosett H L et al (1983) Patterns of Alcohol Consumption and Fetal Development, Obstet Gynecol, 61: 539-546

Royal College of General Practitioners (1974) Oral Contraceptives and Health, London, Pitman Medical Books

Royal College of General Practitioners (1976) The Outcome of Pregnancy in Former Oral Contraceptive Users, Br J Obstet Gynaecol, 83: 608-616

Royal College of Psychiatrists (1985) Drug Scenes A Report on Drugs and Drug Dependence by the Royal College of Psychiatrists, London, Gaskell

Rush, D et al (1980) Diet in Pregnancy: A Randomised Controlled Trial of Nutritional Supplements Birth Defects Original Article Series, 16 (3) New York, Alan R Liss Inc

Ryan, S and Loup, M (1994) Pollution from traffic higher inside cars The Sunday Times 20 March

Rydar, R E J (1993) Natural family planning: effective birth control supported by the Catholic Church BMJ 307; 723-6

Sacks, S L (1986) The truth about Herpes, Vancouver, Verdant Press

Saifer, P and Zellerbach, M (1984) Detox, New York, Ballentine

Salsburg, D See John Elkington

Samarawickrama, G See J Rose

Sandford, M K et al (1992) Neural Tube Defect Etiology: New Evidence Concerning Maternal Hypothermia, Health and Diet, Dev Med Child Neurol, 34: 661-675

Sandstead, H H (1984) Zinc: Essentiality for Brain Development and Function, Nut Today November, December 26-30

Saner, G et al (1985) Hair managanese concentrations in newborns and their mothers, Am J Clin Nut 41: 1042-1044

Sassenath, E N et al (1979) Reproduction in Rhesus Monkeys Chronically Exposed to Delta-9-THC Adv in the Biosciences, 22-23: 501-522

Savage M et al (1973) Maternal varicella infection as a cause of fetal malformations, Lancet, i: 352-354

Scarrel, P M and Pratt, K A (1968) Symptomatic gonorrhea during pregnancy, Obstet Gynaecol 32; 670-673

Schacter, J et al (1979) Prospective study of chlamydial infection in neonates, Lancet, ii; 337-380

Schacter, J & Grossman, M (1983) Chlamydia In: J Remington and J Klein (eds) Infectious diseases of the fetus and newborn infant, WB Saunders & Co

Schafer, C et al (1985) Illness in infants born to women with chlamydial trachomatis infection Am J Dis of Children, 139: 127-133

Schauss, A G (1986) Body Chemistry and Human Behaviour Course at Oxford 18 November

Schelling, J L (1987) Which Drugs should not be Prescribed during Pregnancy, Ther Umsch Rev Ther 441: 48-53

Schmidt, M et al (1993) Beyond Antibiotics, Healthier Options for Families, Berkeley, North Atlantic Books

Schneider, A et al, (1988) Colposcopy is superior to cytology for the detection of early genital human papillovirus infection, Obstet Gynaecol, 71: 236-241

Schoenthaler, S J (1986) Commercial Hair Analysis: Lack of Reference Norms and High Reliability within and between Seven Selected laboratories for 17 Trace Minerals Int J Biosocial Res 1: 84-92

Schroeder, H and Mitchener, M (1971) Toxic Effects of Trace Elements on the Reproduction on Mice and Rats, Arch Envir Health 23; 102

Schofield, C B S (1972) Sexually transmitted diseases, London, Churchill-Livingstone

Schroeder, H A (1973) The Trace Elements and Man, Old Greenwich, Devin-Adair

Schwartz, J et al (1986) Relationship between childhood blood levels and stature, Pediatrics 77(3): 281-283

Seamans, B (1974) In: William Dankenbring

Seidman, D S et al (1992) Birth weight and intellectual performance in late adolescence, Obstet and Gynecol, 79: 545-546

Shapiro, S et al (1976) Perinatal Mortality and Birthweight in Relation to Aspirin Taken During Pregnancy, Lancet, i; 1375-1376

Shephard, T H (1983) Catalogue of teratogenic agents, 4th Edition, John Hopkins Press

Shiota, K (1982) Neural tube defects and maternal hyperthermia in early pregnancy: epidemiology in a human embryo population, Am J Med Gen, 12: 281-288

Shiota, K (1988) Induction of neural tube defects and skeletal malformations in mice following brief hyperthermia in utero, Biology of the Neonate 53: 86-97

Shurygin, G I (1978(The psychogenic pathological development of personality in children and adolescents in families with fathers afflicted with alcoholism, Zhur Nevropat i Psik, 78: 1566-1569

Simpson, J L (1986) Fetal Wastage In; S Gabbe et al, (eds) Obstetrics, Normal and Problem Pregnancies, New York, Churchill-Livingstone

Simpson, J (1957) A preliminary report on cigarette smoking and the incidence of prematurity, Am J Obstet Gynaecol, 73: 800-815

Singh, N et al (1978) Neonatal lead intoxification in a prenatally exposed infant, J Paediat 93(6): 1019-1021

Skreb, N and Frank, Z (1963) Developmental abnormalities in the rat induced by heat shock, J Embryology and Experimental Morphology 11: 445-457

Smith, G A (1947) Effects of maternal undernutrition upon the newborn infant in Holland, J Paediatrics 30: 250-259

Smith, C G and Gilbean , P M (1985) Drug Abuse Effects on Reproductive Hormones In: J Thomas et al (eds) Endocrine Toxicology, New York, Raven Press

Smith, J C et al (1973) Zinc: a trace element essential in vitamin A metabolism, Science, 181: 954-955

Smith, J C et al (1976) Alterations in vitamin A metabolism during zinc deficiency and food and growth restriction, J Nut 106: 569-574

Smith, D W (1979) Mothering Your Unborn Baby, Philadelphia, W B Saunders

Smithells, R W et al (1980) Possible prevention of neural tube defects by preconceptual vitamin supplementation Lancet i: 339-340

Smithells, R W et al (1983) Further experience of vitamin supplementation for the prevention of neural tube defect recurrences, Lancet, i: 1027-1031

Smyth, A (1988) Trouble on Tap, Here's Health, May

Sohler, A et al (1977) Blood Lead Levels in Psychiatric Outpatients Reduced by Zinc and Vitamin C, J Orthomolecular Psychiat 6(3): 272-276

Solletico, D et al (1987) Prenatal chlamydia trachomatis infection with post natal respiratory disease in a preterm infant, Acta Paediat Scan, 76: 932

Soyka, L F and Joffe, J M (1980) Male mediated drug effects on offspring, Prog Clin Biol Res, 36; 49-66

Spatling, L and G (1988) Magnesium supplementation in pregnancy: a double-blind study, Br J Obstet Gynaecol 95: 111-116

Spears, J W S (1984) Effect of Dietary Nickel on Growth, Urease Activity, Blood Parameters and Tissue Mineral Concentrations in the Neonatal Pig, J Nut 114: 845-853

Spivey, Fox M R (1975) New York Acad Science 258: 144

Spyker, J M Occupational Hazards and the Pregnant Worker, Behavioural Toxicology Overview, 470

Stellman, J and Daun, S M (1979) Work is Dangerous to your Health, Vintage Books

Stempak, J G (1965) Etiology of antenatal hydrocephalus induced by folic acid deficiency in the albino rat, Anat Res 151: 287

Stenchever, M A et al (1974) Chromosome Breakages in Users of Marijuana, Am J Obstet Gynaecol, 118: 106-113

Straub, W E (1983) Kepone In: L Parmeggiani (Ed) Encyclopedia of occupational health and safety Vol 1, Int Labour Office, Geneva

Stirling, H F et al (1987) Passive smoking in utero: its effects on neonatal appearance, BMJ 295: 627-628

Stone, D et al (1976) Aspirin and congenital malformations, Lancet, i: 1373-1375

Streissguth, A P (1979) Fetal Alcohol Syndrome: Where are we in 1978? Women and Health, 4; 223-237

Streissguth, A P (1991) What every community should know about drinking during pregnancy and the lifelong consequences for society, Substance Abuse, 12(3): 114-127

Stuttaford, T (1988) Listening In, The Times, 21 July

Stuttaford, T (1994a) Quality of life at birth is in the measure, The Times, 30 August

Stuttaford, T (1994b) A father's lot, The Times, 23 June

Stuttaford, T (1994c) How to have a safe and happy birthday, The Times, 6 December

Suharno, D et al Improvement in vitamin A status may contribute to the control of anaemic pregnant women, Lancet 342: 1325

Sutcliffe, M et al (1993) Prevention of neural tube defects, Lancet 342: 1174

Sutherland, H (1982) Lancet, i

Sutton, G (1982) Genital infections, Midwife, Health Visitor and Community Nurse, 18(2): 42-45

Sutton, G (1988) Personal communication in April

Sutton, G (1991) Paper delivered at FORESIGHT conference in December

Sweetenham, E (1994) An instant test for IVF success ,Observer 22 May

Tarni-Mordi, W (1994) See Wojtas below

Taskinen, H et al (1989) Spontaneous abortions and congenital malformations among the wives of men occupationally exposed to organic solvents, Scandinavian Journal of Work Environment and Health, 15 (5) 345-352

Sutton, G (1988) Personal communication in April

Teymor, M L (1978) Infertility, New York, Grune and Stratton Inc

Thatcher, R et al (1982) Effects of low levels of cadmium and lead on cognitive functioning in children Arch Envir Health 37(3): 159-166

Tomorrow's World (1987) BBC1, 12 November

Tuormaa, T (1994a) The Adverse Effects of Tobacco Smoking on Reproduction, A Review from the Literature, FORESIGHT (Also reprinted in Int J Biosocial Med Res, 14:2)

Tuormaa, T (1994b) The Adverse Effects of Alcohol on Reproduction, A Review from the Literature, FORESIGHT

Turnbull, A C (1984) Amniocentesis In: N J Wald (Ed) Antenatal and neonatal screening, Oxford, Oxford University Press

Turner, G and Collins, E (1976) Fetal effects of regular salicylate intoxification in a newborn, a case report, Clin Pediatr, (Philadelphia) 15: 912-913

Underwood, E J (1977) Trace Elements in Human and Animal Nutrition, New York, Academic Press

US Public Health Service (1980) The Health Consequences of Smoking for Women A Report of the US Surgeon-General, Office on Smoking and Health, US Dept of Health and Human Services, Rockville

US Surgeon General's Advisory on Alcohol and Pregnancy (1981) FDA-Drug Bulletin 11 (12) July

Vallee, B (1965) Zinc In: Comar, C L and Bronner, C S (eds) Mineral Metabolism, Vol II B, London, Academic Press

Van Thiel, D H et al (1975) Alcohol induced testicular atrophy: An experimental model for hypogonadism occurring in chronic alcoholic man, Gastoenterology 69: 326-332

Varma, T R (1987) Infertility, BMJ, 294: 887-890

Vitale, L F et al (1975) Blood lead – an inadequate measure of occupational exposure, J Occ Med 17: 102-3

Von Pirquet, C (1906)

Wald, N J and Bower, C (1994) Folic acid, pernicious anaemia, and prevention of neural tube defects, Lancet 343: 307

Walton, P (1980) New antibiotics in fight against genital disease, Doctor, 11 September, 39

Ward, N I; Durrant, S; Sankey, R J; Bound, J P; and Bryce-Smith, D (1990) Elemental Factors in Human Fetal Development, J of Nutritional Medicine 1, 19–26

Ward, N I (1993) Preconceptual care questionnaire research project, In press Details from FORESIGHT

Ward, N I (1992) Environmental Aspects of Heavy Metals and Aluminium and the Effect on Human Health, FORESIGHT Mid-Summer Newsletter 26-38

Ward, N I et al (1987) Placental element levels in relation to fetal development for obstetrically "normal" births: A study of 37 elements, evidence for effects of cadmium, lead and zinc on fetal growth and smoking as a source of cadmium, Int J Biosocial Res 9(1): 63

Ward, N I (1995) Preconceptual care and pregnancy outcome, J of Nutritional & Environmental Medicine 5, 205-8

Watson, WS et al (1980) Oral Absorption of Lead and Iron Lancet, ii: 237

Webb, T (1984) Reported in: Thomas Stuttaford The screen of fear, The Times 15th November

Weber, L W D (1985) Benzodiazepines in pregnancy – academic debate or teratogenic risk? Biol Res in Preg, 64: 151-167

Webster, W S and Edwards, M S (1984) Hyperthermia and the induction of neural tube defects in mice, Terat, 29: 417-425

Wertheimer, N and Leeper, E (1984) Adverse effects on fetal development associated with sources of exposure to 60 hz electric and magnetic fields (Abstract), 23rd Hanford Life Sciences Symposium Interaction of Biological Systems with Static and ELF Electric and Magnetic Fields, Richland, W A

Wesselhoeft, C and Pearson, C M (1950) Orchitis in the course of severe chickenpox with pneumonitis, followed by testicular atrophy, N Eng J Med 242: 651

West, Christine P (1987) Age and infertility, BMJ 294: 853

Westrom L (1975) Affect of acute pelvic infectious disease on fertility, Am J Obstet Gynecol, 121: 707-713

Wetherall, C F (1981) Kicking the Coffee Habit, Minneapolis, MN

Whorton,MD et al(1977) Infertility in male pesticide workers, Lancetii:1259-61

Wibblerley, D G et al (1977) Lead levels in human placentas from normal and malformed births, J Med Gen 14(5): 339-345

Wichit, S and Bracken, M B (1985) Caffeine consumption during pregnancy and association with late abortion, Am J Obstet Gynecol, 154; 14-20

Wichman, L (1992) The value of semen analysis in predicting pregnancy, Acta Universitatis Tamperensis Ser A, Vol 34: 6:5

Williams III, J et al (1992) Chorion Villus Sampling: Experience with 3016 Cases Performed by a Single Operator, Obstet Gynaecol, 80: 1023-1029

Williams, R J (1956) Biochemical Individuality: the basis for the genetotrophic concept, New York, Wiley

Williams, R J (1973) Nutrition Against Disease, London, Bantam

Williams H (1969) The Pill in New Perspective: Pregnant or Dead? San Francisco, New Perspective Publications

Wilson, G S et al (1979) The development of preschool children of heroin addicited mothers: a controlled study, Pediat, 63: 135-141

Winston, R M L (1986) Infertility, A Sympathetic Approach, Martin Dunitz Ltd

Witkin, S S (1985) Infections in Modern Medicine, 129-132

Woffinden, B (1994) Cows: mad or poisoned? Living Earth and The Food Magazine, 184:10

Wojtas, O (1994) Clues cut risks of early birth, Times Higher Educ Sup 4 Feb

Wolff, H et al (1991) Chlamydia trachomatis induces an inflammatory response in the male genital tract and is associated with altered semen quality, Fert Ster 55(5): 1017-1019

World Health Organisation (1981) A prospective multicentre trial of the ovulation method of natural family planning 1 The teaching phase, Fert Ster 36; 152-8

Wright et al (1978) Neoplasia and dysplasia of cervix uteri and contraception: a possible protective effect of the diaphragm, Br J Cancer 38: 273-279

Wright, P (1988) Claims that power cables cause Cancer to be investigated, The Times, 18 March

Wynn M and Wynn A (1981) The Prevention of Handicap of Early Pregnancy Origin, London Foundation for Education and Research in Childbearing

Wynn A and M (1986) Prevention of Handicap of Early Pregnancy Origin Today – Building Tomorrow International Conference on Physical Disabilities, Montreal, 4-6 June

Wynn A and M (Undated) Should Men and Women Limit Alcohol Consumption when Hoping to have a Baby? London, The Maternity Alliance

Yale, W et al (1985) Teachers' ratings of children's behaviour in relation to blood lead levels, Br J Dev Psych 2: 285-306

Ylikahri, R et al, (1974) Hangover and testosterone, BMJ, 2:445

Young, R (1984) Pesticide found in a third of fresh fruit, The Times, 16 April

Yudkin, J (1986) Pure, White and Deadly, London, Viking

Ziff, S (1985) The Toxic Time- Bomb, Wellingborough, Thorsons

INDEX